ERRATA

IMPORTANT – Please note the following changes to the text:

page 8, Table 2.1 under *'Children'*

   for   'Triclofos (Tricloryl)   250 mg kg^{-1}'
   read 'Triclofos (Tricloryl)   25 mg kg^{-1}'

page 16, 2nd column, 2nd paragraph, 3rd line

   for   'maldevelopment of the upper jaw'
   read 'maldevelopment of the lower jaw'

page 34, Table 5.2, under column headed *'Agent'*

   for   'Propofol (Ativan)'   *read* 'Propofol (Diprivan)'

page 55, 2nd column, 6th line
   for   '900 mmHg . . .'   *read* '90 mmHg . . .'

Page 67, 2nd column, under heading **'(a) Inspiratory phase'**, line 5
   for   'is usually limited to about 0.6 kPa or 60 cmH$_2$O'
   read 'is usually limited to about 6 kPa or 60 cmH$_2$O'

page 110, 2nd column, under heading **'Technique'**, line 1
   for   'A 20 or 22 G cannula . . .'
   read 'A 23 or 22 G cannula . . .'

page 128, 2nd column, under **'(b) Pulmonary function tests'**, line 1
   for   'Vital Capacity (VC) . . . . . . ml kg^{-1} l'
   read 'Vital Capacity (VC) . . . . . . 70 ml kg^{-1} '

A NEW SHORT TEXTBOOK OF
ANAESTHETICS, INTENSIVE CARE AND PAIN RELIEF

NEW SHORT TEXTBOOK SERIES

Some titles in the series

A New Short Textbook of Surgery
Leonard Cotton
Kevin Lafferty

A New Short Textbook of Microbial and Parasitic Infection
B. I. Duerden
T. M. S. Reid
J. M. Jewsbury
D. C. Turk

A NEW SHORT TEXTBOOK OF
ANAESTHETICS, INTENSIVE CARE AND PAIN RELIEF

JOSE PONTE
MD, PhD, FFARCS

Senior Lecturer and Honorary Consultant Anaesthetist,
King's College Hospital School of Medicine and Dentistry, London

DAVID W. GREEN
MB, BS, FFARCS

Consultant Anaesthetist, King's College Hospital
School of Medicine and Dentistry, London
and Deputy Director, Intensive Care Units, King's College Hospital
and Dulwich Hospital, London

HODDER AND STOUGHTON
LONDON SYDNEY AUCKLAND TORONTO

To Carmo, George and Monica, whose support
and practical help kept me going, and
to my father
JCP

To my family
DG

British Library Cataloguing in Publication Data
Ponte, Jose C.
 A new short textbook of anaesthetics,
 intensive care and pain relief.
 1. Anesthesia
 I. Title   II. Green, David W.
 617'.96   RD81
ISBN 0 340 37681 3

(International Student Edition)
ISBN 0 340 41031 0

First published 1986

Typeset and printed in Great Britain
by Page Bros (Norwich) Ltd
for Hodder and Stoughton Educational
a division of Hodder and Stoughton Ltd, Mill Road
Dunton Green, Sevenoaks, Kent

Contents

Foreword

There are many today who would like to know something about anaesthesia, and the question is often asked 'What will succinctly give me a comprehensive account of modern anaesthetic practice?' Ponte and Green have attempted to produce just such a manual. The authors are acknowledged teachers from an eminent Department of Anaesthetics of one of London's great Teaching Hospitals (King's College Hospital). Their approach is novel in that they cover ground not attempted before in any 'Introduction to Anaesthesia'. Starting with a short historical review, they outline the principal features of anaesthetic equipment and drugs, followed by an account of specialised anaesthesia and the common mishaps. It is all very clear and sensible teaching. The authors then continue with a section on Intensive Care and another on the Treatment of Chronic Pain, all of which encompasses the growing field of anaesthetic knowledge. A most welcome introduction at the end is an appendix outling the principles of pharmacology related to anaesthesia and also a most useful self-assessment questionnaire. This is fun for the reader and in keeping with the modern popularity of Multiple Choice Questions.

As this book is very readable, it is also good teaching, and will find favour with students and all those interested in anaesthesia. I think the authors have achieved their objective and I wish them well with their new enterprise.

H. C. Churchill-Davidson

Preface

This book has evolved from our experience of teaching medical students and junior anaesthetists at King's. The shorter texts presently available, we found, were either out of date, limited in contents or inadequately pitched for the requirements of our students and first year SHOs.

The book was designed primarily to teach only the rudiments of anaesthetic practice and aspects of general medicine in which anaesthetists have unique expertise. There are chapters on applied physiology and pharmacology, as the review of such subjects is highly appropriate in the context of anaesthesia and intensive care. The importance of these topics is generally recognised, but hard to find in books written at this level.

Those embarking on an anaesthetic career may well find this book a useful 'starter' in the first year of training. The practical nature of the contents may also be useful to other trainees such as house surgeons, and nurses undertaking further training in anaesthetics, intensive care and recovery.

We are indebted to Dr T. D. W. Davies for his comments and suggestions during the preparation of this book. Our thanks also go to Christopher Allen for the time he put into reading the manuscript and providing us with constructive comments from the viewpoint of a medical student.

J. C. Ponte and D. W. Green

1

Survey of anaesthetic techniques; historical notes

The purpose of anaesthesia is to render the patient temporarily unconscious or insensitive to pain so that operations or diagnostic/therapeutic procedures can take place comfortably.

This 'end product' can be obtained in three different ways:

General anaesthesia
Regional anaesthesia
Other methods (e.g. hypnosis, acupuncture)

The proportion of procedures carried out under general anaesthesia varies considerably from country to country, and in the UK varies between hospitals.

The belief that regional anaesthesia is safer than general anaesthesia is not supported by the national figures of morbidity and mortality caused by anaesthesia, perhaps because a number of regional anaesthetics are given by practitioners without specialised training in anaesthesia and resuscitation.

For most operations below the waist and on the upper limbs a choice can be made between general and regional anaesthesia. Intrathoracic, upper abdominal, head and neck operations are usually carried out under general anaesthesia.

General Anaesthesia

The administration of a general anaesthetic is often compared to flying an aeroplane. The pilot carefully inspects his machine just prior to flying, and the flight comprises three phases: take off, level flight and landing. A general anaesthetic comprises the same number of steps:

Pre-anaesthetic assessment/ premedication	Pre-flight check
Induction	Take off
Maintenance	Level flight
Recovery	Landing

Induction of anaesthesia simply means rendering the patient unconscious and unreactive to surgical stimuli. This is usually achieved by intravenous injection of a powerful drug called an induction agent, of which thiopentone is an example. In children, due to greater difficulty with venous access, an inhalation induction is frequently achieved with the aid of nitrous oxide and a volatile anaesthetic agent like halothane.

During maintenance the patient is kept anaesthetised for as long as the operation lasts by inhalation of nitrous oxide supplemented by either an inhalational agent or intravenous narcotic analgesics plus a neuromuscular blocker.

Recovery starts at the end of the operation and lasts until the patient is fully conscious and able to resume all physiological functions affected by the anaesthetic. Most complications of anaesthesia are seen during induction and recovery.

Various techniques of general anaesthesia can be employed depending on individual circumstances.

(a) Without intubation of the trachea

The patient breathes the mixture of anaesthetic gases and vapours delivered to the airway via a face mask; this technique is suitable for most minor surgery.

(b) With intubation of the trachea

A plastic or rubber tube is passed through the mouth (occasionally the nose) into the trachea, after a neuromuscular blocker has been administered intravenously. The gaseous anaesthetic is then delivered through the tube. This technique is mandatory for ENT, eye or dental operations under general anaesthesia, because of the difficulty of effectively maintaining a patent airway without interfering with surgery. Intubation is also required whenever artificial ventilation must be used. Provided long-acting neuromuscular blockers or high doses of analgesics are not given, most anaesthetics can be carried out with the patient breathing spontaneously.

(c) With intermittent positive pressure ventilation (IPPV)

This is mandatory when long-acting neuromuscular blockers are used for intra-abdominal or intrathoracic operations. Intubation of the trachea is always required. IPPV can be produced by manually squeezing a bag or by means of a ventilator (Chapter 10).

There are several other techniques that form part of the repertoire of an experienced anaesthetist; for example, a neuromuscular blocker may not be required for the type of operation performed but the anaesthetist chooses to use it in conjuction with nitrous oxide and a narcotic analgesic for maintenance of general anaesthesia. This is described as 'balanced anaesthesia', usually the most suitable for patients with cardiac disease. In general terms all induction and volatile agents have depressant effects on the cardiovascular system which are dose dependent. This has been identified as being due to a direct effect upon the myocardium and indirectly by reducing sympathetic tone. Some analgesic agents like fentanyl and neuromuscular blockers like pancuronium are almost devoid of these depressive effects. A maintenance technique based on these two agents is usually preferred in patients with poor cardiac function.

Regional Anaesthesia

A number of techniques fall into this category (Chapter 18), such as:

(a) *Conduction anaesthesia*, including peripheral nerve blocks, epidural and spinal anaesthesia.

    (1) Peripheral nerve blocks. All the major peripheral nerves and plexuses of the upper and lower limbs can be blocked by percutaneous techniques. A small gauge needle is inserted through the skin until the tip lies within the sheath of the neurovascular bundle. Then a local anaesthetic agent is injected, such as 1.5% lignocaine. The larger the nerve the larger the volume needed; both sensory and motor conduction are blocked. Brachial plexus blocks are frequently used, but individual nerves in the upper limb are less frequently blocked, and those in the lower limb even less. Intercostal nerve blocks are widely used, and are very useful in the management of chest trauma with fractured ribs.

    (2) Epidural analgesia or anaesthesia. This consists of injecting local anaesthetic into the epidural space between the dura and the bone. Lumbar interspaces are most frequently used (lumbar epidural), but the sacral hiatus (caudal epidural) or the thoracic spaces (thoracic epidural) are also used.

    (3) Spinal analgesia or anaesthesia. Local anaesthetic is injected into the subarachnoid space through a thin needle. Spinal anaesthesia has a rapid onset (5 min) compared with epidural (20–40 min). Most surgery below the waist can be carried out under spinal or epidural anaesthesia.

(b) *Infiltration and surface blocks*
Usually carried out by the surgeon; the local anaesthetic solution is injected into the tissues surrounding the lesion or the incision, or directly applied to the epithelium (eye, nose, mouth, urethra and skin).

(c) *Intravenous block* (Bier's block)
Local anaesthetic solution is injected intravenously via a small cannula inserted into a

distal vein of the upper limb, having applied a tourniquet proximally. Anaesthesia of the limb follows within 5–10 minutes and is effective for as long as the tourniquet is inflated. Surgery of the forearm can be carried out using this technique; certain chronic pain conditions are often relieved by injecting in this way a local anaesthetic mixed with a vasodilator (Chapter 18).

Historical Notes

The choice of techniques outlined above has not always been available. For example, only 35 years ago few anaesthetists were experienced in tracheal intubation, and muscle relaxants were not routinely used. Automatic ventilators were just being introduced into what were to become the first intensive care units (ICU).

In 1800, Sir Humphrey Davy, who had made extensive studies on nitrous oxide, suggested that it might be useful to soothe the pain of surgical operations.

There are important landmarks in the history of anaesthesia that are also relevant to medical history generally:

(a) The first convincing demonstration of a general anaesthetic was given by W. T. G. Morton, using ether, at the Massachusetts General Hospital in 1846.

(b) The first spinal anaesthetic was conducted by A. K. G. Bier in 1898 in Kiel, and the first epidurals were conducted in Paris around 1901 independently by Cathelin and Sicard.

(c) Landsteiner described the major blood groups (ABO) in 1901. This allowed successful compatible transfusion in man to become commonplace. Citrate was first used as an anticoagulant in 1914, and blood banks were established in Russia (Moscow), and the USA (Mayo Clinic, Rochester and Cook County, Chicago) in the 1930s.

(d) Thiopentone, the first acceptable intravenous agent, was introduced by J. S. Lundy in 1934 in the USA, and is still the most popular induction agent throughout the world.

(e) Manually controlled breathing during anaesthesia was introduced in 1940 by Guedel and Nosworthy. Tubocurarine was introduced to enhance muscle relaxation by Griffith and Johnson of Montreal in 1942. It was used for a few subsequent years in small doses (up to 10 mg) with the patient breathing spontaneously. Only later were larger doses (e.g. 45 mg) and intermittent positive pressure ventilation (IPPV) used.

(f) The Copenhagen polio epidemic in 1952 stimulated the development of artificial ventilation by IPPV in Denmark and Sweden. This event contributed to the setting up of the first ICUs. Björk and Engström described IPPV for post-operative respiratory failure in 1955.

(g) Halothane was used clinically for the first time, by Johnstone of the Manchester Royal Infirmary, in 1956. It is still the most popular volatile agent in the western world.

Pre-operative management: assessment and premedication

Pre-operative Assessment

The aim of pre-operative assessment is to assess the risks of surgery and anaesthesia, and to balance them against the benefits of the proposed operation. It must therefore be jointly carried out by the surgeon and anaesthetist concerned.

The houseman or medical student clerking the surgical patient should be the first to detect and draw attention to the abnormalities likely to cause problems with anaesthesia. The following areas should be covered systematically and note be made of:

General Aspects

(a) Complicated previous anaesthetics or history of specific anaesthetic problems in the family: e.g. absence of plasma cholinesterase or an undetected myopathy causes problems with suxamethonium.
(b) Smoking causes an increase in the incidence of post-operative pulmonary complications. Blood levels of carbon monoxide found in smokers, cause a reduction in oxygen carrying capacity equivalent to the loss of $2\,g\,dl^{-1}$ of Hb.
(c) Drinking habits, drug abuse, long-standing sedative or analgesic therapy increases anaesthetic requirements.
(d) Obesity is a serious obstacle to anaesthesia partly for mechanical reasons like intu-

bation, turning and tilting of the patient, and also because of the increased demand upon the heart and respiratory muscles. Finding suitable veins is difficult.
(e) Dehydration or hypovolaemia make induction and maintenance of anaesthesia very hazardous (Chapter 6). It must always be corrected prior to anaesthesia with appropriate intravenous infusions.

Anaemia and Bleeding Disorders

Long-standing anaemia is well tolerated; chronic renal failure patients often present with Hb values as low as $6\,g\,dl^{-1}$. In acute anaemia the compensatory increase in cardiac output is usually inadequate; Hb should be brought up to $10\,g\,dl^{-1}$ by specific therapy in elective cases, or by transfusion of packed red cells in emergencies. Haemoglobinopathies, especially sickle cell disease, should be treated before anaesthesia by blood transfusion until the level of Hb-S falls to less than 30% of total. Sickle cell trait does not require pre-operative treatment, but throughout anaesthesia and recovery a higher fraction of inspired oxygen ($FIO_2 > 0.4$) should be used.

Bleeding disorders are more a surgical than an anaesthetic problem. Pre-operative transfusion of concentrates of the missing factor is indicated (Chapter 6).

Drugs

A few drugs interact adversely with anaesthetic agents (Chapter 5). Most regular medication should be given in the usual dosage right up to the last pre-operative hour, with a few exceptions:

(a) Oral antidiabetic agents should be stopped 2 days pre-operatively because of the risk of hypoglycaemia due to their prolonged action.
(b) Antidepressants of the monoamine oxidase inhibitor group, now rarely used, should be stopped 2 weeks pre-operatively because of their adverse interaction with analgesics and other anaesthetic agents. Lithium salts should be stopped 3 days pre-operatively because they may unpredictably potentiate neuromuscular blockers.
(c) Warfarin should be stopped at least 24 hours pre-operatively, and prothrombin time checked. It should be in the region of 1.6–2:1 with reference to control. If it exceeds 2:1 the operation should be postponed until this level is reached, but in an emergency fresh frozen plasma may be administered together with a small dose of vitamin K. If necessary change over to a heparin infusion to maintain anticoagulation. The effects of warfarin may be enhanced or reduced by many of the anaesthetic and analgesic agents, by alteration of plasma protein binding and liver inactivation.

The anaesthetist must be aware of all other medication taken by the patient. Amongst the most important are:

(a) Corticosteroids if given for more than 6 weeks, because of possible adrenocortical (and hence cardiovascular) depression.
(b) Antihypertensive agents, including beta-blockers, because the regulation of the blood pressure is altered, particularly in response to blood loss.
(c) Central analgesic and sedative drugs, because their chronic use stimulates liver metabolism with consequent shorter duration and effect of anaesthetic agents.

Cardiovascular System

Congenital or acquired valvular disease, and ischaemic heart disease are all important. This is usually apparent in the history and examination, but only a few elements are significantly correlated with cardiac risk at operation. Some important ones are:

(a) History of myocardial infarction in the previous six months. If possible, the operation should be postponed.
(b) Evidence of heart failure, such as dyspnoea, basal crepitations, ankle swelling, increased jugular venous pressure or gallop rhythm.
(c) Any form of dysrhythmia, and in particular more than five ventricular ectopic beats per minute.
(d) Hypertension, especially if untreated, and angina pectoris.

Some of these factors are reversible with treatment, and this must be done before the operation unless it is an emergency. Supraventricular dysrhythmias in young patients must always be investigated and pre-operative anti-dysrhythmic treatment instituted.

Regional anaesthesia is not safer than general anaesthesia in patients with cardiovascular disease.

Respiratory System

Chronic respiratory disease is justifiably worrying for the anaesthetist.

(a) Asthma

Intractable bronchospasm ranks high in the list of contributory causes of death under anaesthesia. Long-term bronchodilator therapy should be continued right up to operation: e.g. a salbutamol inhalation may be given with premedication. Antihistaminic agents such as promethazine and oral theophylline may be added to the premedication. The anaesthetic must be conducted with careful avoidance of all drugs and mechanical stimulation known to trigger bronchospasm. Avoid endotracheal intubation if possible. Intravenous atropine effectively prevents vagal reflexes; beta-blockers, even if beta-1 selective, must not be used.

(b) Chronic airways disease

The seriousness of the situation is easily assessed by asking how far can the patient walk without shortness of breath, or asking the patient to count numbers in one single expiration. The number of previous hospital admissions related to the respiratory condition is important.

If the maximum uninterrupted walk is less than 50 metres, or the patient is unable to count up to 10 in a single breath, or there has been more than one hospital admission due to respiratory disease, then pulmonary function tests, including blood gas analysis, should be requested.

If the forced expiratory volume at one second (FEV_1) is less than 50% of FVC and the latter less than 50% of predicted, blood gas analysis must be done. The post-operative course is best correlated with the resting PaO_2 and $PaCO_2$ values when breathing air. Three degrees of severity may present, with different post-operative prognoses:

(1) $PaO_2 > 7.3$ kPa   (55 mmHg)   and   normal $PaCO_2$: reasonable prognosis
(2) $PaO_2 < 7.3$ kPa and normal $PaCO_2$: absolute need of special post-operative care and possibly mechanical ventilation
(3) $PaO_2 < 7.3$ kPa   and $PaCO_2 > 6$ kPa (45 mmHg): very poor prognosis, and almost certain to need prolonged post-operative ventilation.

Chronic respiratory patients benefit from regional anaesthetic techniques if suitable for the operation. If general anaesthesia must be given, competitive neuromuscular blockers (NMB) should be kept to a minimum, because the smallest interference with respiratory muscles often leads to severe respiratory failure.

Neuromuscular Disease

(a) Myopathies

Myotonic syndromes cause a generalised con-tracture in response to suxamethonium. Responses to competitive NMBs may be either decreased or abnormally prolonged.

(b) Myasthenia gravis

The use of competitive NMBs is usually contra-indicated; a normal dose can cause incapacitating paralysis for more than 48 hours. Post-operatively the patient must be managed in the ITU.

Diabetes

Diabetic patients fall into one of three classes: those managed on diet alone, those on oral anti-diabetic drugs, and those on insulin. They are all at an increased risk in surgery because of the vascular and neurological changes associated with the disease.

In minor (non-stressful) surgery only patients on insulin or oral therapy require special management, mainly because of the fasting period surrounding the operation. Antidiabetic tablets should be stopped 48 hours prior to surgery to reduce the risk of hypoglycaemia. Patients on long-acting insulin should be switched over to soluble insulin 12 hours pre-operatively. The normal regime should be re-established as soon as the patient is able to eat. Frequent checks of blood glucose will need to be made.

All diabetic patients need special attention to insulin demands in major surgery because stress increases insulin requirements (partly due to release of catecholamines). A 5% dextrose drip should be instituted pre-operatively and a constant infusion of soluble insulin started. The hourly rate of insulin administration should initially be based on the individual daily requirements, and adjusted at two or four hour intervals depending upon blood glucose levels. This regime should be continued during the operation, and post-operatively until the patient has recovered from operative stress and resumed a normal diet. Two- or four-hourly measurements of blood glucose must be taken during this period, so that hypo- or hyper-glycaemia are rapidly corrected.

Others

(a) Renal failure

Patients with renal disease may present with difficult anaesthetic problems, e.g. severe anaemia, high plasma potassium and prolongation of drug effects. Volatile agents such as halothane or isoflurane, mostly eliminated through the lung, are good choices. If competitive NMBs must be used, atracurium or vecuronium are preferred.

(b) The liver

The liver poses surprisingly few problems to the anaesthetist, except in end-stage liver failure. It is only then that the elimination of drugs, normally metabolised in the liver, is affected. A very rare form of necrotising hepatitis has been reported in some patients in association with repeated exposure to halothane.

(c) Anatomical deformities

In particular those of the jaw or the chest; the first because of difficulty with tracheal intubation and the second because of extra demand upon the respiratory muscles (e.g. kyphoscoliosis).

(e) Epilepsy

This is not a contraindication for anaesthesia; most antiepileptic agents enhance the ability of the liver to metabolise anaesthetic drugs, therefore increasing demand. Anticonvulsant treatment is continued right up to the time of premedication and restarted as soon as is practicable (i.m. or oral) post-operatively.

(f) Pregnancy

Only emergency surgery should take place. Thiopentone, suxamethonium, pancuronium, pethidine and halothane are examples of safe, well-tried agents that may be used in early pregnancy. After the 16–18th week the risk of regurgitation of stomach contents at induction increases steeply, and the same precautions should be taken as for caesarean section (Chapter 8).

Assessment Scale

The American Society of Anesthesiologists (ASA) has produced a classification of patients depending on their general condition before operation. This scale bears some correlation with morbidity and mortality due to operation or anaesthetic, and is useful as a means of recording and conveying to others the state of the patient:

ASA I   Normal healthy patient
ASA II Patient with mild systemic disease
ASA III Severe systemic disease limiting normal activity
ASA IV Incapacitating systemic disease which is a constant threat to life
ASA V   Moribund, not expected to survive 24 hours with or without operation
E—Signifies that the operation is to be performed as an emergency. Generally speaking this places the patient in the next highest risk category.

Premedication

Premedication is a traditional measure thought to be necessary for all patients undergoing surgery. It has its roots in the days of gaseous induction with ether which caused intense salivation and production of tracheal secretions. With modern anaesthetic techniques anti-sialagogues are rarely necessary, and the main purpose of premedication is to relieve anxiety.

Indications

The indications for premedication are to:

Relieve anxiety
Produce sedation and amnesia
Reduce secretions
Relieve pain
Modify the autonomic response to induction of anaesthesia

(a) Anxiety

Anxiety is not shared by all patients in anticipation of an operation, and reassurance is often as effective as medication. Benzodiazepines are specifically indicated to suppress anxiety, but a mixture of an opiate with hyoscine or a phenothiazine is similarly effective.

(b) Sedation and amnesia

Sedation is usually desirable in children, and can be obtained with trimeprazine, promethazine, triclofos or diazepam. Amnesia is sometimes desirable in adults when the events surrounding the operation are particularly unpleasant; benzodiazepines or hyoscine are effective.

(c) Secretions

Secretions rarely interfere with surgical procedures, except saliva in oral surgery. Neonates and small children form a special group, which is more susceptible to excessive tracheobronchial secretions due to the small calibre of upper airways. Atropine, hyoscine or glycopyrronium are indicated. An unpleasantly dry mouth is the commonest side effect of these agents; hyoscine and to a lesser extent atropine cross into the brain, exerting a depressant effect that can be excessive in the elderly and the very young (glycopyrronium does not cross the blood–brain barrier).

(d) Pain

Patients are rarely in pain before elective operations. If present, a central analgesic is indicated.

(e) Autonomic response to induction of anaesthesia

The cardiovascular system reflects the autonomic responses to anaesthetic drugs and to intubation of the trachea. Intubation causes the most dramatic changes, with hypertension and tachycardia occasionally requiring the use of blocking drugs; bradycardia with hypotension due to a vagal reflex is uncommon. Pre-operative beta-blockade may be indicated in patients with ischaemic heart disease or intracranial space occupying lesions.

(f) Antiemesis

An antiemetic is usually included with opiate premedication to reduce the incidence of nausea associated with these drugs (Chapter 5).

Examples of Premedications

Examples of premedications are given in Table 2.1.

TABLE 2.1

Average adults (doses in mg)	*males* (70 kg)	*females* (60 kg)	*route*
(a) Papaveretum (Omnopon)	20	15	i.m.
Hyoscine (Scopolamine)	0.4	0.3	1 h pre-op.
(b) Diazepam (Valium) or	10	10	oral
Lorazepam (Ativan) or	2	2	2 h pre-op.
Temazepam	20	20	
Elderly (>65)			
Pethidine	50–75	50–75	i.m.
Atropine	0.6	0.6	1 h pre-op.
Asthmatics			
Pethidine	75–100	50–75	i.m.
Promethazine (Phenergan)	25	25	1 h pre-op.

Children (oral doses, 2 hours pre-operatively)
Trimeprazine (Vallergan) 4 mg kg^{-1}
Diazepam (Valium) 5 mg (if over 20 kg b.w.)
Triclofos (Tricloryl) 250 mg kg^{-1}

i.m. – intramuscular injection; pre op. – pre-operatively; b.w. – body weight

Dehydrated or hypovolaemic patients require smaller doses. The very sick or those for emergency operations are best left unpremedicated.

The anaesthetic machine; gas delivery systems for resuscitation

The Anaesthetic Machine

The anaesthetic machine commonly in use is also known as the Boyle's machine, after the first design by Boyle in 1917. The basic configuration is seen in Fig. 3.1, and is held by a frame on wheels, usually carrying 2 oxygen and 2 nitrous oxide cylinders; these are connected via special fool-proof (pin-index) fittings to reducing valves which maintain pressure in the pipes at 410 kPa (4 kg cm^{-2} or 60 p.s.i.). These high pressure pipes are connected to adjustable needle valves leading to gas flow meters known as rotameters (a rotating bobbin 'floats' in the gas stream within a graduated glass pipe). Each rotameter is calibrated for one gas only. The outlet of the rotameters join together into a wider bore pipe, where the gases mix, leading to the patient's airway. Interposed between rotameters and patient are several devices in the following order:

(1) One or more vaporisers, designed to add volatile agents (e.g. halothane, enflurane) to the gas stream;
(2) Overpressure safety valve which blows off at 30 kPa (305 cmH$_2$O);
(3) Oxygen by-pass system which allows oxygen to flow directly between the high pressure pipe and the outlet of the machine, by operating a press-button or a lever. Anaesthetic gases and vapours are automatically cut off.

The following points must be emphasised for the safe operation of the machine:

(a) Where piped gases (O$_2$ and N$_2$O) at 410 kPa (4 kg cm^{-2} or 60 p.s.i.) are installed, a special connector leading directly to the rotameters through a one-way valve is available in the back or side of the machine.
(b) Pressure gauges are installed in most machines (in some only for the oxygen supply) which read values inside the cylinders, giving an idea of reserve available.
(c) In addition to oxygen and nitrous oxide, most machines in Britain also have similar valve/rotameter systems for 2 more gases, carbon dioxide and cyclopropane. They mix with the main stream at the same point.
(d) All new machines, and most now in use, have an audible device that operates when the pressure in the oxygen pipe drops below 400 kPa. This warns the anaesthetist of exhaustion of the oxygen cylinder in use or of a lack of pressure in the outside supply.
(e) The flow of gases in the rotameters is read with accuracy only when the bobbin rotates freely; readings should be taken from the top edge of the bobbin.
(f) When operating the machine always turn oxygen on first and off last; always ensure that one oxygen cylinder is full at the start of each anaesthetic and that the vaporisers are all turned off.
(g) The outlet of the machine can be connected

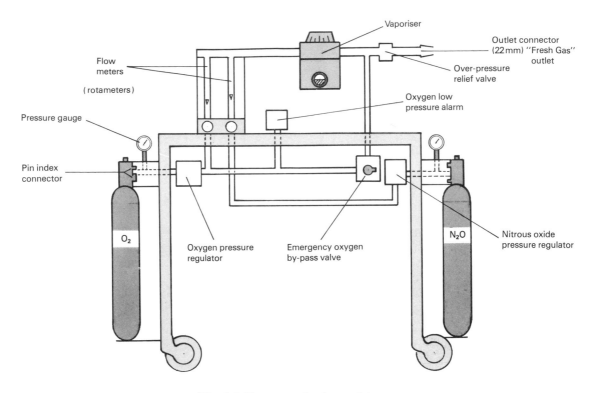

Fig. 3.1 The anaesthetic machine

to a variety of gas delivery systems or ventilators; always ensure that a pressure to inflate the lungs can be generated at the outlet of the machine: e.g. by filling a rubber bag with gas having closed the expiratory valve and blocked the outlet of the delivery system with the finger. On squeezing the bag it should be evident whether the system is gas-tight or leaky.

In addition to the Boyle's machine there are other types of anaesthetic machine designed to be used under special circumstances, e.g. when pressurised gases are not available.

Vaporisers

Vaporisers (Fig. 3.2) are precision instruments designed to produce accurate concentrations of anaesthetic vapours within a wide range of gas flows $(0.3{-}20\,l\,min^{-1})$. Each vaporiser can be used with one type of volatile agent only, and must be kept vertical to maintain accuracy.

Most designs are based on a variable bypass arrangement. This means that part of the flow through the vaporiser is diverted into a chamber where it is saturated with the anaesthetic vapour and then mixed in precise proportions with the main stream of gas. Temperature compensation devices are fitted to the bypass regulator of most vaporisers, maintaining constant concentrations of vapour at the outlet in spite of cooling due to heat of vaporisation. The majority of vaporisers are designed to operate on the anaesthetic machine, interposed between rotameters and outlet, because they present a considerable resistance to gas flow; some models have been designed to operate within an anaesthetic circuit or a draw-over type of system where gases are propelled by the patient's breathing. These must present very little resistance to gas flow.

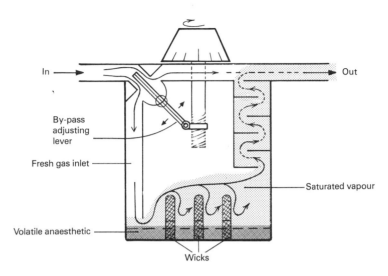

In

Out

By-pass
adjusting
lever

Fresh gas inlet

Saturated vapour

Volatile anaesthetic

Wicks

Fig. 3.2 Schematic drawing of a variable bypass vaporiser

Many anaesthetic machines in use have an additional vaporiser fitted (clear glass bottle with a plunger) designed to be used with ether or trichloroethylene. The concentration of anaesthetic delivered is inaccurate and they have fallen into disuse as a result.

Gas Delivery Systems

The set of tubes, valves, reservoir bag and soda lime containers attached to the outlet of the anaesthetic machine is the 'anaesthetic breathing system'; it is often designated as the 'anaesthetic circuit', although a circuit of gases is rarely present. Commonly the 'circuit' is absent and a ventilator is inserted between anaesthetic machine and patient.

There are basically two types of system in use: rebreathing systems with carbon dioxide (CO_2) absorption in which the patient rebreathes most of the expired gas, and the non-rebreathing systems in which most of the expired gases are wasted.

(a) Rebreathing or 'circle' system

This consists of a container with soda lime (CO_2 absorber) connected by a rubber tube to the outlet of the anaesthetic machine, through which the 'fresh gas' is delivered. At the top of the absorber two corrugated rubber tubes lead to the face mask or endotracheal tube where they join in a Y or T piece, as shown in Fig. 3.3a. The gas flow within these tubes is unidirectional due to valves fitted at the absorber end. The gas returned from the patient is delivered to the bottom of the absorber such that it flows through the soda lime in an upward direction. The designation of 'circle' system is due to this unidirectional flow of gases. Soda lime comprises a mixture of calcium hydroxide (95%) and sodium hydroxide (5%). Although carbon dioxide is absorbed by calcium hydroxide the reaction is too slow without the addition of sodium hydroxide. The latter combines rapidly with carbon dioxide forming sodium carbonate which then transfers the carbon dioxide to calcium hydroxide. As a result, sodium hydroxide is reformed and the overall reaction may be simplified to:

$$Ca(OH)_2 + CO_2 \longrightarrow CaCO_3 + H_2O$$

A colour indicator warns of impending soda lime exhaustion. One kg of soda lime absorbs approximately 20 l of carbon dioxide.

A spring-loaded valve, fitted to the absorber, allows escape of excess gas; this valve can be

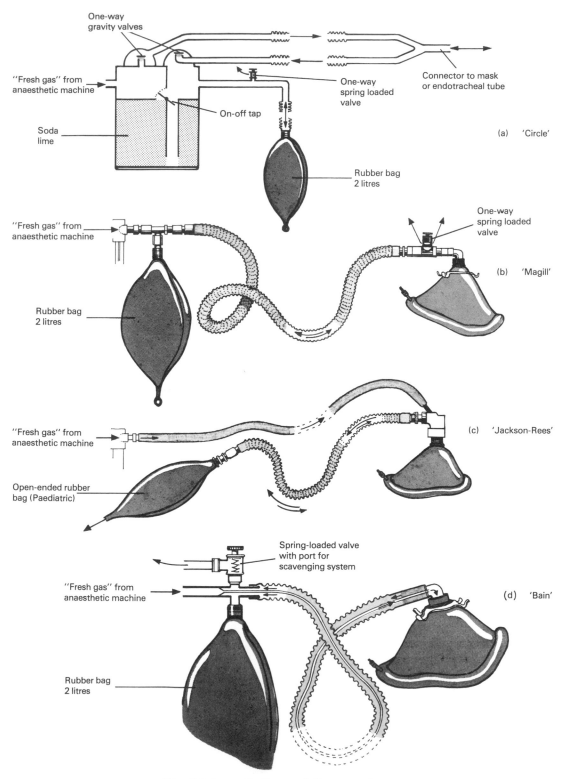

One-way
gravity valves

"Fresh gas" from
anaesthetic machine

Soda
lime

On-off tap

One-way
spring loaded
valve

Connector to mask
or endotracheal tube

(a) 'Circle'

Rubber bag
2 litres

"Fresh gas" from
anaesthetic machine

One-way
spring loaded
valve

(b) 'Magill'

Rubber bag
2 litres

"Fresh gas" from
anaesthetic machine

(c) 'Jackson-Rees'

Open-ended rubber
bag (Paediatric)

Spring-loaded valve
with port for
scavenging system

"Fresh gas" from
anaesthetic machine

(d) 'Bain'

Rubber bag
2 litres

Fig. 3.3 Anaesthetic gas delivery systems

partially closed to apply pressure to the airway if necessary. Another length of corrugated tube, with a two litre rubber bag at the end, is fitted to the inspiratory end of the absorber; the bag gives an indication of the patient's tidal volume or may be used for positive pressure ventilation (Fig. 3.3a).

Most CO_2 absorbers are provided with a lever operating a bypass to the soda lime permitting its renewal without interrupting the circuit.

Advantages of the circle system are:

(1) economy in running, necessitating much smaller fresh gas flows than non-rebreathing circuits;
(2) preservation of humidity and temperature of respired gases; and
(3) reduced amount of anaesthetic gases and vapours escaping and polluting the atmosphere of operating theatres.

Disadvantages of the circle system are:

(1) difficulty in predicting concentrations of anaesthetic vapours inhaled by the patient.
(2) inconvenience of having to replace exhausted soda lime; and
(3) bulky and impractical to clean and sterilise.

(b) Non-rebreathing systems

There are a variety of configurations depending on whether the fresh gas flow arising from the anaesthetic machine is delivered close to the patient's airway, and where the reservoir bag and expiratory valve are placed. Figure 3.3 depicts the schematic arrangement of the most commonly used systems in modern practice. As long as the fresh gas flow is adequate to prevent rebreathing of expired CO_2, any of the systems may be used for all purposes, spontaneous or assisted ventilation, adult or paediatric. Each system has its own minor advantages when used by experienced practitioners. Lightness of weight, provision for collection of expired and excess gases to reduce pollution, and ease of cleaning are obvious advantages.

Basic Systems for Resuscitation

Emergency positive pressure ventilation can be delivered without any apparatus, as mouth to mouth or mouth to tube ventilation. The two most commonly used devices to provide emergency ventilation are:

(a) Self-expanding bag with three-way valve (Fig. 3.4a)

This consists of a 2 litre rubber or plastic bag which returns to orginal shape after squeezing. A one-way valve is fitted at one end of the bag, and a special three-way valve is attached at the opposite end. The latter may be connected to a face mask or endotracheal tube. The three-way valve operates as shown in Fig. 3.4; gas may only flow from bag to patient or from patient to atmosphere. The function of the valve is the same whether the patient breathes spontaneously or positive pressure is applied. This system is portable and does not require compressed gases or other external sources of power, but simply the hand of the operator. Oxygen, if available, may be added to the bag via an accessory inlet.

(b) Rubber bag, T-piece, valve and oxygen cylinder (Fig. 3.4b)

This arrangement is perhaps the most commonly available in hospital wards. The flow of oxygen is set at about 10 l min by turning the knob on the flowmeter; time must be allowed for filling of the bag and the valve (Heidbrink valve) must be partially closed to prevent the escape of gas and enable the operator to generate a pressure in the airway of the patient. If attached to an endotracheal tube there is little difficulty in adjusting the aperture of the valve. If a face mask is used, the commonest problem encountered is lack of adequate seal around the edge of the mask. In inexperienced hands this may be very frustrating; a higher oxygen flow (e.g. $15–20 \, l \, min^{-1}$) may lead to a slight improvement.

Checking of Apparatus

Finally, all apparatus used in anaesthesia and

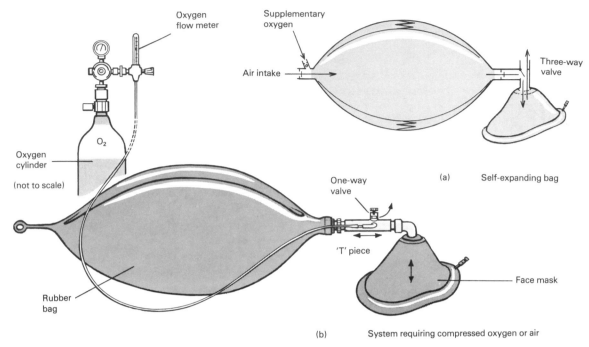

Fig. 3.4 Emergency gas delivery systems. (a) Self-expanding bag (e.g. 'Ambu' bag), not requiring compressed oxygen or air source. Oxygen can be added if available. (b) 'Waters' type system, requiring a source of compressed oxygen or air

resuscitation should be checked at regular intervals and again just prior to use.

The following points must be checked:

(a) Oxygen supply in the anaesthetic machine

Ensure that there is an oxygen supply (always start with one reserve cylinder full) connected to the appropriate flowmeter. This is done by turning on the oxygen flow and then closing the oxygen valve on the cylinder (or disconnecting the pipe from the building supply); the flowmeter reading should fall to zero and the audible alarm should be triggered. Reconnection of the supply should restore flow in the rotameter. All the other gases supplied in the machine should be checked in the same way (except for the alarm).

(b) Vaporisers

Check that vaporisers contain anaesthetic, the dials move, and are all turned off.

(c) Leaks in gas delivery systems

Check that the gas delivery system has no leaks and a pressure can be generated in the bag by closing all valves and blocking the patient outlet with a finger. Check for perished rubber and blocked pipes.

Gas Cylinders—Colour Code

Gas	Shoulder	Body
air	Black/white	black
oxygen	white	black
nitrous oxide	blue	blue
entonox	blue/white	blue
carbon dioxide	grey	grey
cyclopropane	orange	orange

4

Practical aspects of anaesthesia: airway, drips and monitoring of blood pressure and electrocardiogram

Maintenance of the Airway: Care of the Unconscious Patient

Introduction

Maintenance of a clear airway is of crucial importance during anaesthesia and intensive care. Respiratory obstruction, usually due to the tongue falling back onto the pharynx, is the major cause of morbidity and mortality during general anaesthesia particularly in the recovery phase. The principles employed to avoid this problem in the perioperative period are applicable in other emergency situations such as following drug overdose, airway trauma and cardiac arrest.

Recognition of Airway Obstruction

Airway obstruction in the conscious patient is easily recognised as it leads to strenuous efforts on the part of the patient to overcome it. However, the unconscious patient may not exhibit classical compensatory signs when obstructed. One sees paradoxical chest move-

ment, where the upper abdomen and chest see-saw during attempted inspiration, the chest retracting and the abdomen sticking out. Lack of air entry and exit means that air movement cannot be detected by listening at the mouth, and obviously the patient will eventually become cyanosed. Application of a bag and mask (e.g. Waters circuit) and observation of bag movement provides conclusive proof.

Sites and Treatment of Respiratory Obstruction

See also Chapter 11 and Fig. 4.1

(a) Nasal passages

Although the nasal passages are the 'normal' portal for air from atmosphere to lungs, obstruction does not usually cause problems as air may equally well pass via the buccal cavity. However, neonates are inveterate 'nose breathers' and do not adopt mouth breathing easily, even when the nasal airway is totally obstructed, e.g. from choanal atresia. Insertion of an oral airway and placement of the infant in the prone position may allow temporary respite, but often surgical

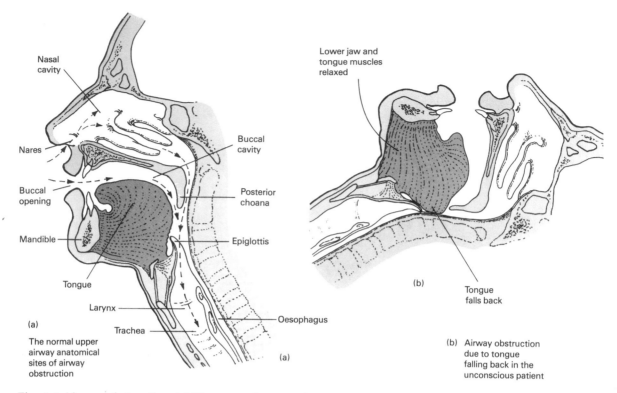

Fig. 4.1 Airway obstruction (a) The normal upper airway: anatomical sites of obstruction; (b) obstruction due to tongue falling back in the unconscious patient

relief of the obstruction is necessary as an emergency.

(b) Buccal cavity

By far the commonest cause of obstruction in the mouth is relaxation of the jaw muscles due to anaesthesia or any central nervous system depressant (e.g. head injury, alcohol, benzodiazepines). The tongue falls back onto the posterior wall of the pharynx thus preventing air passage (Fig. 4.1b). Luckily this is also the easiest form of obstruction to treat. In the anaesthetised patient, the lower jaw is mechanically lifted forwards taking the tongue with it and thus clearing the airway. This manoeuvre may be combined with insertion of an oral airway which mechanically interposes itself between the pharynx and the tongue (Fig. 4.2). The patient who is unconscious from other causes or has a full stomach, should be turned on to the side with a head down tilt. Not only does this

usually 'automatically' clear the airway by allowing the tongue to fall away from the pharynx, but should vomiting occur, it is much less likely to be aspirated. All unconscious patients should be recovered on their sides.

Other causes of airway obstruction in the mouth are much less common. In the neonate, maldevelopment of the ~~upper~~ *lower* jaw with a large tongue pushing back against the pharynx (e.g. Pierre Robin syndrome) causes respiratory obstruction which may need urgent treatment. The tongue is stitched and pulled forward, and the baby nursed prone. Trauma to the buccal cavity may lead to mechanical obstruction, e.g. by teeth, dentures or oedema of the tongue and pharynx which prevents free passage of air. Apart from the general measures mentioned above, endotracheal intubation may be required. Infectious causes in the mouth and pharynx, e.g. Ludwig's angina and retropharyngeal abscess, cause obstruction by swelling. Foreign bodies, especially vomitus, should

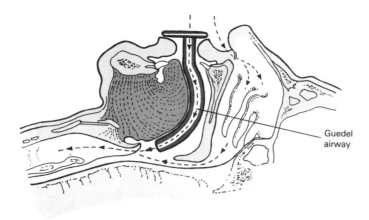

Guedel
airway

Fig. 4.2 Re-establishment of patent airway by insertion of
oral (Guedel) airway

always be sought for and cleared manually in
suspect cases.

(c) Epiglottis, larynx and trachea

Infective causes are mentioned in Chapter 11.
Sudden obstruction is commonly due to trauma
or foreign body aspiration, especially particulate
matter in vomitus. If this cannot be removed
manually or by instrumentation through the
mouth, cricothyrotomy or tracheotomy may be
necessary to bypass the obstruction. Below the
level of the trachea, blockage of air passages
does not produce complete obstruction so is not
dealt with further here.

Special Techniques

(a) Endotracheal intubation (ETI)

As mentioned in Chapter 11, relief of airway
obstruction by the methods outlined in Section
IVb may only provide temporary relief prior to
definitive ETI. To accomplish this skilfully and
atraumatically requires considerable practical
experience. The practice of some 500 endotracheal intubations is the minimum that most
anaesthetists in training need to feel reasonably
confident. This is usually accomplished in the
first six months of training. There is great varia-

bility in the anatomy of the region, so unex-
pected difficulties arising in this manoeuvre are
not uncommon.

As a life-saving measure, non-anaesthetists
have a better chance of effectively providing
respiratory support with a bag and mask (and
airway if needed), than unsuccessfully attempting to place an endotracheal tube. Turning the
patient on the side and head down, with careful
observation and frequent suction of the
oropharynx is usually adequate to prevent gross
inhalation of stomach contents. Whilst preparations are made, it is important that the airway
is maintained by other means as outlined above,
and the patient fully oxygenated.

Equipment selection (Fig. 4.3)
The following will be required:
   A pressurised source of oxygen and gas delivery system
   Mask and airway of suitable size (a mask size
   of 3 or 4 with a size 2 Guedel airway is
   suitable for female adults, with one size
   bigger for males)
   A cuffed endotracheal tube (ETT) for oral use
   (these are numbered according to their
   internal diameter in mm. A size 8 is suitable
   for females and 9 for males. In the emergency situation smaller sized tubes should
   be available)

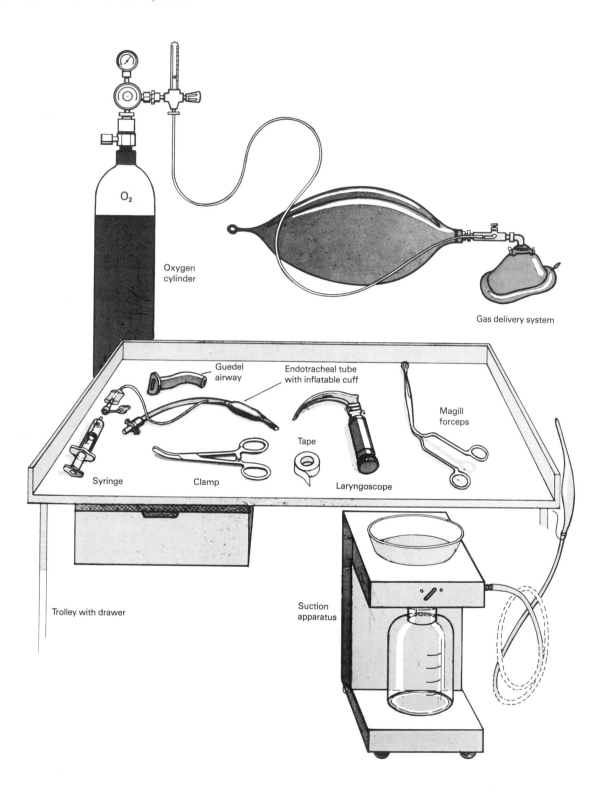

Fig. 4.3 Endotracheal intubation trolley

A laryngoscope of appropriate size (A Macintosh size 3 or 4 for adults)

A syringe and clamp for cuff inflation, ties, etc.

Intubating forceps (Magill) for guiding the ETT and also for removing foreign bodies

Drugs (Chapter 5)

A good suction apparatus

Technique

The patient is turned onto the back and a pillow placed underneath the head. This flexes the neck so that the chin is directed towards the chest. The head is then extended by pulling back on the chin towards the operator. This 'sniffing the morning air' position is designed to align the planes of the mouth with that of larynx (Fig. 4.4). The mouth is opened by separating the lips and pulling on the upper jaw and lip with the index finger. The laryngoscope is held in the left hand, and enters the mouth with the blade directed towards the right tonsil. On reaching this level, the blade is swept to the midline, keeping the tongue on the left, and out of sight. At this point the epiglottis comes into view. The blade is gently advanced until it reaches the angle between the base of the tongue and epiglottis. It is important to get the earliest view of the epiglottis and not lose sight of it, so as to avoid going too far and misinterpreting the oesophagus for the larynx. At this stage the whole laryngoscope is lifted upwards and away from the operator so that the larynx comes into view. This may also require pressure on the trachea just below the cricoid ring to produce optimal alignment (Fig. 4.4b).

The ETT is taken in the right hand with the inner curve of the tube facing the right side of the mouth so as to minimally impede the view of the larynx as the tube is inserted. If possible, observe the tube entering the larynx and push it in only until the cuffed portion disappears beyond the cords. This avoids inadvertent endobronchial intubation. The cuff is inflated to provide an airtight seal and the bag squeezed to ascertain correct placement of the tube by listening to both sides of the chest with a stethoscope.

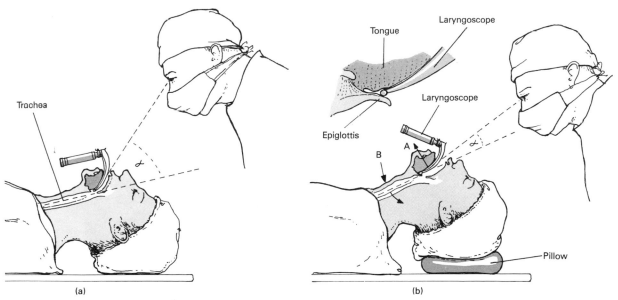

(a)   (b)

Fig. 4.4 Principles of visualization of larynx with laryngoscope prior to endotracheal intubation. (a) Shows the patient in an incorrect position prior to attempted intubation. The greater the value of angle 'alpha', the greater the difficulty in visualising the larynx, particularly if the neck is not flexed. (b) Shows the correct position with the neck flexed on a pillow and the head extended ('sniffing the morning air'). Angle 'alpha' is now minimal, especially if gentle traction is exerted on the laryngoscope in the direction shown (A), and the larynx rotated on its axis by pressure below the cricoid cartilage (B). It is easy to see that the laryngeal and visual planes are now more closely aligned

(b) Cricothyrotomy and tracheotomy

In extremely rare circumstances, e.g. anatomical abnormalities, foreign body lodged in larynx, epiglottis, endotracheal intubation may be impossible. Nevertheless, an airway must be established urgently. The technique of cricothyrotomy is one that should be learned as it is almost always preferable to tracheotomy in the emergency situation where a skilled operator and the necessary instruments are not to hand.

Equipment

Special apparatus for cricothyrotomy is manufactured but infrequently available. A compromise is often made such that oxygenation is maintained via one or more large bore intravenous cannulae (e.g. 12 or 14G) whilst preparations are made for definitive tracheotomy. The luer connection of the cannula can be attached to an anaesthetic gas delivery system via a sawn off 2 ml syringe and catheter mount. Oxygen may be blown down the cannula intermittently, which is usually sufficient for metabolic demand, but CO_2 elimination will be inadequate.

Technique

The cricothyroid membrane must be located between the thyroid cartilage and cricoid ring in the midline anteriorly. It may help maximally to extend the neck with a pillow underneath the shoulders. The needle and cannula combination are then inserted through the membrane, the needle removed and the cannula connected as described above. In extreme circumstances where no specialised equipment is available, an ordinary penknife can be inserted through the membrane, and any improvised tube (e.g. empty biro) used to enlarge the hole (Fig. 4.5).

The formal technique of tracheotomy is beyond the scope of this text.

Other Aspects of Care of Unconscious Patients

Regardless of the cause, unconsciousness means that the protective reactions to pain and discomfort are absent. Circumstances permitting, the patient should be put on the side with a slight head down tilt (e.g. following a grand mal convulsion).

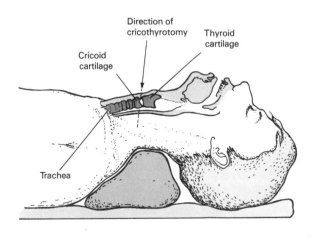

(a)

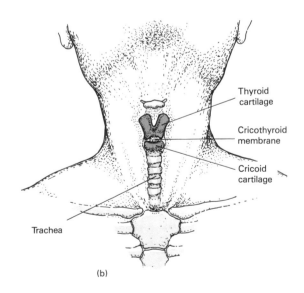

(b)

Fig. 4.5 Anatomical landmarks for performing cricothyrotomy. (a) Shows the lateral view of the patient lying flat with a pillow under the shoulders. (b) Shows the anterior view of the cricothyroid membrane through which the cricothyrotomy is performed. Note the landmarks on either side, the thyroid and cricoid cartilages. The cricothyroid membrane forms a shallow depression between them

The cornea of the eye may dry and suffer irreversible damage due to absence of tears and blinking; so, eyes should be taped closed during unconsciousness.

Shoulder and hip joints should be protected from pulling and excessive passive movement to prevent dislocation.

Peripheral nerves may suffer prolonged compression or stretching, so watch out for hard, sharp edges pressing on the lateral surface of the leg (superficial peroneal nerve) or the side of the face (facial nerve). The brachial plexus is perhaps the most vulnerable to stretching and compression due to over-extension of the arm or by keeping the patient in the lateral position without additional support under the rib cage.

Maintenance of body temperature is important. Wet garments must be replaced soon after surgery and the patient kept well covered with blankets if ambient temperature is below 24°C. During prolonged major surgery a warming blanket should be used.

Finally, remember that the unconscious patient should be turned in bed or trolley at regular intervals of 30 minutes to relieve effects of pressure on the skin, and great care must be exercised not to drop the unconscious patient on the floor on transferring to or from bed!

Setting up an Intravenous Infusion

This is best learnt by doing it. Beginners should practice the whole sequence many times over, starting with unwrapping the giving set, the bag of intravenous fluid and the cannula; the proper practice of connecting the three parts without contamination and the presence of air bubbles can only be learnt by watching an experienced person first and then doing it under supervision (Fig. 4.6). The practice of some 50 cannulations is perhaps the minimum required to feel some confidence with the technique (or to give it up!).

Only short-term cannulation will be discussed. Long-term cannulation (weeks rather than days) is best done through a large deep vein (subclavian or internal jugular), with rigorous aseptic conditions, by an experienced person.

Venous cannulation is best practised initially in anaesthetised patients. In awake patients any cannula bigger than 22G should not be inserted without anaesthetising the skin to be punctured with a small amount of 1% lignocaine through a 25G needle.

(a) Choice of vein

The first important step is to choose the appropriate vein for the purpose. Except in very special circumstances, only the superficial veins of forearm and hand should be used. The areas of the wrist and elbow should be avoided because this requires splinting of the joint and there is an increased likelihood of the cannula becoming dislodged or the vein thrombosed. A 'Y' junction in the forearm is probably the best choice for beginners, because the entry into the vein is more obvious (Fig. 4.7).

(b) Choice of cannula

There is no evidence that different makes of cannula has any influence upon the success of peripheral vein cannulation. Of the presently available models perhaps only cost should be considered in the choice (Fig. 4.8).

Depending upon the objective in mind, the appropriate size of cannula should be chosen. Table 4.1 is a guide for the usual applications

TABLE 4.1 Choice of i.v. cannula

Application	Internal diameter mm	Gauge SWG	Max. flow rate ml min^{-1}
Continuous infusion of drugs (pumped)	0.8–1.0	22–20	25–50
Normal daily fluid replacement	1.2	18	65
Slow blood transfusion or intraoperative fluids	1.7	16	150
Rapid blood transfusion	2.0–2.4	14–12	200–300

SWG – Standard wire gauge.

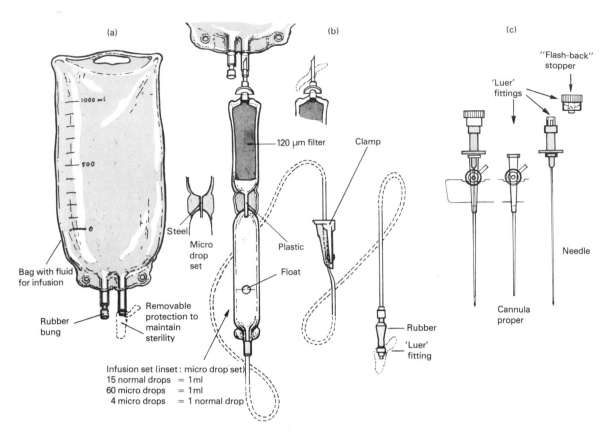

Fig. 4.6 Essential components to set up a drip. (a) Bag with fluid for infusion; (b) infusion set (inset: microdrop set); (c) intravenous cannula, showing components

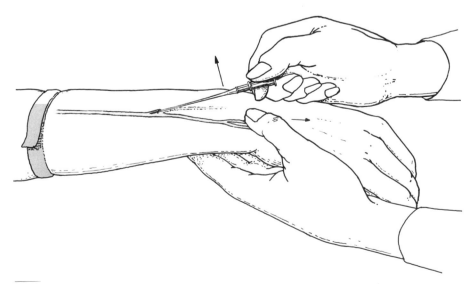

Fig. 4.7 Insertion of cannula into vein. Arrows indicate direction of pull

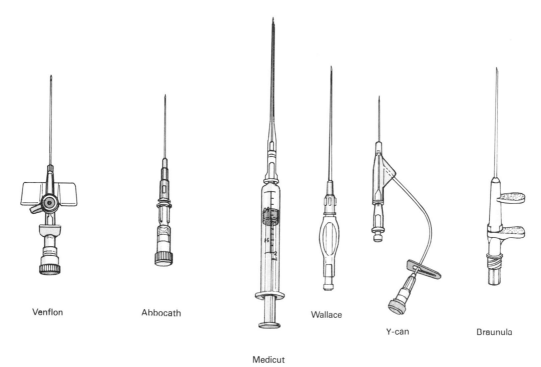

Venflon   Abbocath   Wallace   Y-can   Draunula

Medicut

Fig. 4.8 Examples of available intravenous cannuli

(c) Preparation of insertion site

A tourniquet, blood pressure cuff or a helpers hand must be placed proximal to the puncture site to distend the vein. The pressure applied round the arm must be such that blood flow in the arteries is not compromised (check for radial pulse if in doubt). If vein distension is insufficient, gently tapping it at a rate of $3–4\,s^{-1}$ for 1 minute, or application of a warm towel for 2–3 minutes, usually produces a rewarding improvement.

The operator must wash his hands before starting the procedure, but the value and techniques of disinfecting the site of puncture are much debated. If a disinfectant is used (alçohol, chlorhexidene or iodine-based preparations) at least 1 minute should be allowed for it to take effect prior to puncture.

Shaving of the skin produces small abrasions which alter the skin flora, and should be done only to facilitate the application of adhesive tape.

(d) Technique of insertion

The left hand of the operator holds the patient's arm (or hand) steady, the thumb pulling the skin taut, distally to the puncture site, without collapsing the vein. With the bevel of the needle facing upwards, the cannula/needle assembly is advanced through the skin a few mm from the vein, using a quick jabbing action, at an angle of approximately 20 degrees to the surface of the skin. Note that the assembly must be held by the hub of the needle and not by the hub of the cannula. The cannula is then further advanced until it enters the vein with a feel of a 'click' followed by flash-back of blood into the hub. It is then advanced some 3–5 mm inside the vein, the needle pulled out some 10 mm and the whole assembly advanced until the cannula is fully inserted (Fig. 4.7).

(e) Fixation of the cannula and maintenance of flow

There is an infinite variety of methods of securing the cannula to the skin. Good common sense is the most important factor. Even the most perfect way of taping the cannula *in situ* is easily defeated by a moist or greasy skin.

If the drip is to be used in the awake patient over a few days, it is worth spending a bit more time in devising a firm way of securing the cannula in place. The important aspects of the technique preventing accidental removal of the cannula are (Fig. 4.9):

- The tensile strength of the tape (depends on width)
- The adhesiveness of the tape (depends on type)
- The area of adhesive surface in contact with dry skin and with the cannula
- The direction of the tape applied on the skin with respect to the cannula
- Presence of hair
- Shielding of the giving set from potential sources of pulling

The important factors in preserving the patency of the drip are those that prevent thrombosis and infection. The longer the length of cannula inside the vein the higher the incidence of thrombosis; cannuli placed at the wrist or elbow tend to cause thrombosis more rapidly due to trauma to vein wall. Injection of drugs through the drip increases the chances of thrombophlebitis; the irritant action of drugs and hypertonic or acidic solutions has the same effect.

Daily dressing of the puncture site and the use of local antiseptic agents is mandatory. In some hospitals in other European countries (but not the US) the routine practice of inserting a new cannula in a different site every 24 hours (also changing the giving set and fluid container) has been found to be cost effective.

At the first signs of local inflammation the cannula must be removed and replaced elsewhere, preferably in the other arm.

Measurement of Arterial Blood Pressure

Introduction

Techniques based upon inflation of an arm cuff are by far the commonest; recently a number of automated devices based on similar principles have been introduced with great success.

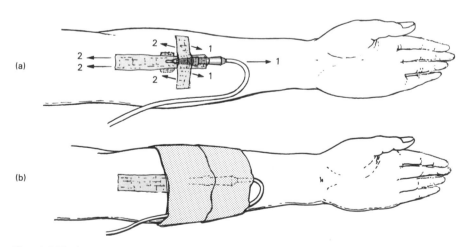

Fig. 4.9 Technique of securing cannula and drip set to the arm. (a) First step. Arrows indicate direction of forces which may act to pull cannula out (1) and to keep cannula in place (2). A wide adhesive tape (25 mm) is preferable at this stage; the distal end of the longitudinal piece is rolled round the hub of the cannula for maximum adhesiveness. (b) Second step. The whole area should be covered with wide (6–10 cm) elastic tape or bandage to stabilise the tube of the giving set and preventing the loop from being accidentally caught

In special circumstances direct measurement via an indwelling arterial cannula may be necessary, such as in cardiac, neuro and major vascular surgery, hypotensive anaesthesia and in the critically ill patient.

(a) Indirect methods

(1) *Sphygmomanometry*

The principle of operation of the sphygmomanometer is usually well taught in medical basic sciences courses and in general nursing courses. Figure 4.10 will suffice to refresh the memory. If a stethoscope is used an estimation of both diastolic and systolic pressures is possible, because of the sudden drop in turbulence as the pressure in the cuff becomes less than diastolic. By finger palpation of the radial artery, systolic pressure can be estimated and the value will be some 5–10 mmHg lower than that obtained with the stethoscope.

It should be remembered that sphygmomanometry is only an indirect estimation of blood pressure.

(2) *Oscillotonometry*

Anaesthetists tend to prefer this method in the operating theatre since it does not require a stethoscope. It is also based upon the principle of inflating a cuff round the arm above the systolic blood pressure and allowing its pressure to drop slowly.

The instrument in fact has two cuffs, proximal and distal, within the same wrapping. The proximal cuff has the same function as in the sphygmomanometer; the distal one is used as a sensitive pressure detector (Fig. 4.11a). The instrument has a large dial with a pointer connected to either of two aneroid capsules, and is calibrated in mmHg. Normally the pointer reads the pressure in the proximal cuff, but by pressing a lever on the side of the instrument it reads pressure in the distal cuff. Initially, both cuffs are inflated above systolic pressure, and then let down slowly.

When the pressure in the proximal cuff is above systolic, no variations are seen in the distal cuff. As soon as the pressure drops below systolic, the pointer will show oscillations in the

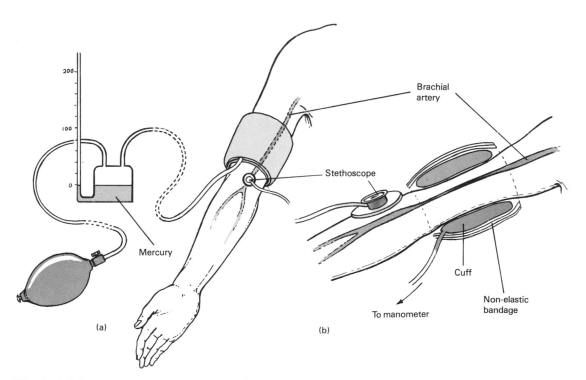

Fig. 4.10 Sphygmomanometer. (a) General arrangement of the mercury manometer and cuff; (b) effect of inflating the cuff upon the artery

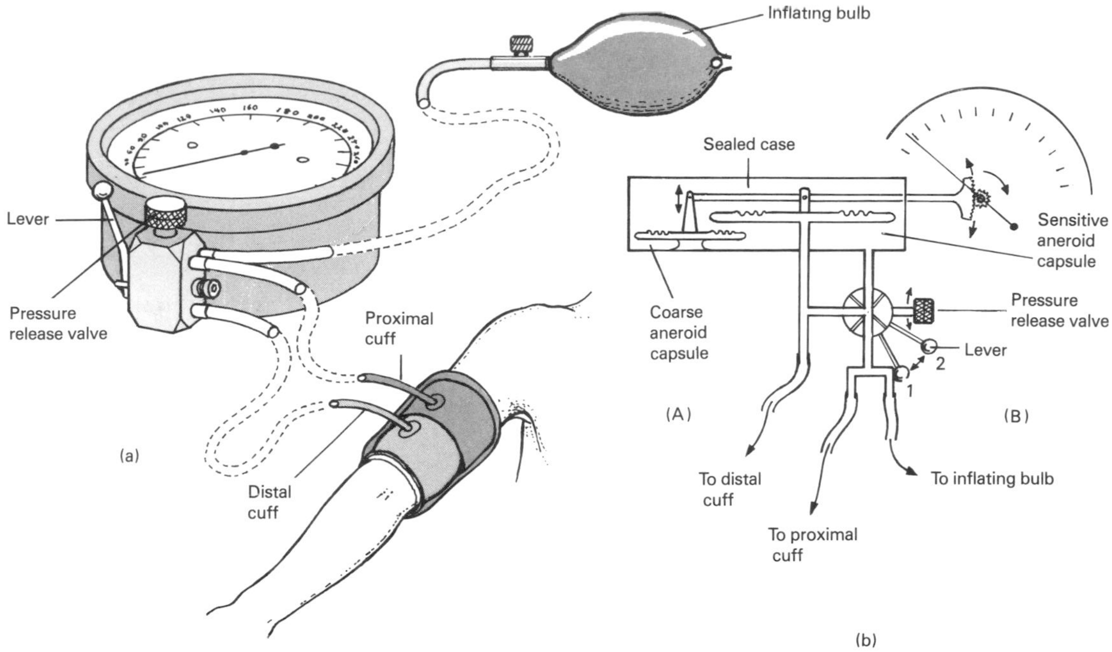

Fig. 4.11 Oscillotonometer of Von Recklinghausen. (a) General arrangement showing the correct connections for cuffs and inflating bulb. (b) Schematic drawing showing the operation of the instrument. Two aneroid capsules (A and B, inside the sealed case of the instrument) operate a lever mechanism, connected to the pointer by a 'rack and pinion' converter. Capsule A is sealed, and capsule B is connected to the distal cuff. With lever in position 1 (as shown) the release valve is cut off, and there is free communication between the two sides of capsule B and the instrument case. On pumping the system, pressure rises equally in both cuffs and inside the sealed case of the instrument: the pointer moves up due to depression of capsule A (capsule B unchanged). On moving lever to position 2 a narrow aperture is interposed between the two sides of capsule B, and the release valve can be used to reduce pressure gradually. Pulsations occurring in the distal cuff are transmitted to the inside of capsule B only (the lever moves at its fulcrum)

distal cuff produced by the momentary distension of the collapsed brachial artery, with each systole. On reaching diastolic pressure, the size of the oscillations is suddenly reduced because the artery is no longer collapsed during diastole (Fig. 4.11b).

(b) Direct methods

These require the insertion of a cannula into a peripheral artery, usually the radial. The cannula is then connected to a length of plastic tubing primed with heparinised saline, connected at the other end to a measuring device. If only mean arterial pressure is required a simple aneroid manometer may be used. If systolic and

diastolic pressure values and information about the shape of the pressure waveform are needed, a pressure transducer must be used. This method also allows for alarm systems to be built in (Fig. 4.12).

Monitoring the ECG in Anaesthesia

(a) Introduction

In the last 5 to 10 years, ECG monitoring during anaesthesia has become routine, even for minor operations in healthy patients. Patients with pre-existing cardiac disease and ECG changes

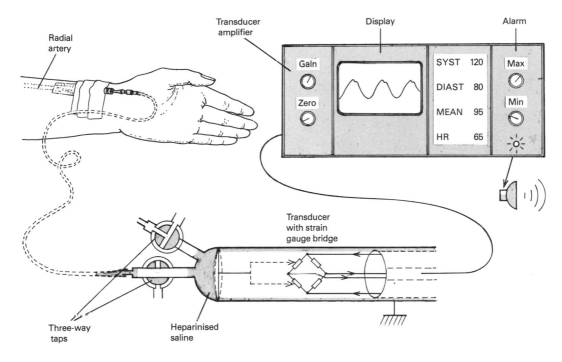

Fig. 4.12 Pressure transducer, bridge amplifier, display and alarm

obviously benefit from ECG monitoring, but what changes and abnormalities can be detected from its use in the previously fit patient? First, it is necessary to consider apparatus and lead placement.

(b) Apparatus and lead placement

The conventional 12 lead ECG is obtained using an electrocardiograph from which a printed record is obtained for analysis. For 'real time' monitoring during anaesthesia and in the intensive care unit (ICU) an oscilloscope is used on which the electrical signal from the heart is directly displayed. Many units also employ 'memory' devices which enable abnormalities to be stored and separately displayed using a 'freeze' and 'cascade' facility. For permanent records, a separate printer is necessary, although these are not routinely available in theatre.

It would obviously be inconvenient to place electrodes on every anaesthetised patient to allow a full 12 lead record to be obtained. Indeed, most theatre monitors are only equipped for 'bipolar' electrodes (3 lead systems) and not

those necessary for the augmented or chest leads obtainable from the 12 lead ECG. There is also, usually, no provision for lead selection. In addition, frequent movement and contact with the patient by the surgical and anaesthetic team has necessitated the use of 'filters' which cut out spurious noise and movement artifact, even including diathermy suppression in the more sophisticated units. Although the signal obtained is clearer, there is an unfortunate tendency for it to be degraded, and as a result, the ECG, particularly the ST segment changes (indicative of ischaemia, see below) are more difficult to interpret. Switching the filters off is possible in some units by changing from the 'monitoring' to the 'diagnostic' mode.

With only three leads available, it is important that lead placement is optimised to produce the most useful information. The bipolar leads involve measurement and display of the difference in electrical potential (from the heart) between two points on the body surface. Conventionally, the three limb leads are utilised, I II and III. 'I' measures the difference in potential between right arm and left arm, 'II' right arm and left leg, 'III' left arm and left leg. The 3 leads include two that are 'active', and one that is 'inactive' (earth). The former two may be placed to record leads I, II or III, the inactive lead being placed anywhere on the body surface. However, the information which primarily needs to be obtained relates to dysrhythmia and ischaemia detection.

Whilst lead II is useful for the diagnosis of supraventricular dysrhythmias, none of the three bipolar leads is really suitable for detection of ischaemia. With regard to the conventional 12 lead ECG, it has been found that about 90% of detectable ischaemic changes are present in lead V5. Although this cannot be measured directly with a 3 lead ECG, a modified V5 (CM5) system can be employed (Fig. 4.13a). This involves placing one active lead (usually designated 'right arm') on an electrode over the upper right of the sternum, and the other ('left arm') on an electrode placed in the usual V5 position (6th intercostal space under the left nipple). The inactive lead is usually placed on the left shoulder. This CM5 configuration not only produces a modified V5 record for ischaemia detection, but also is excellent for dysrhythmia monitoring as it is aligned in the same direction as lead II. One also notes, in practice, that the amplitude of the signal is greater in this position (as one electrode is over the left ventricle), allowing for the gain (and also the noise) of the ECG amplifier to be reduced.

(c) Dysrhythmia detection

(1) Supraventricular dysrhythmias occur frequently in normal anaesthetised subjects, but are rarely dangerous. The sino-atrial (SA) node is particularly susceptible to shielding or suppression by halothane, especially if the arterial carbon dioxide tension ($PaCO_2$) is also low. This results in a junctional rhythm with absent or abnormal P waves (Fig. 4.13b). Sinus bradycardia frequently follows vagal stimulation (such as from pulling on the mesentery or intra-

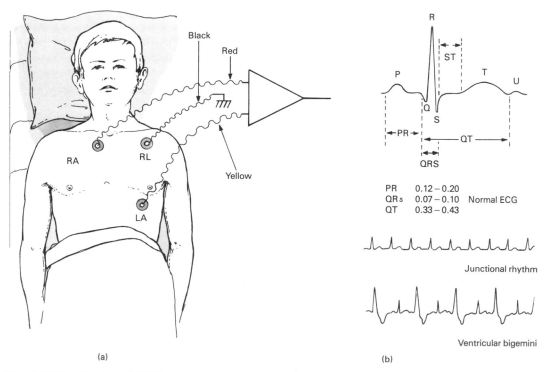

(a)   (b)

Fig. 4.13 Monitoring of ECG during anaesthesia and in intensive care. (a) CM5 configuration of leads. (b) The normal ECG and examples of two common dysrhythmias

ocular manipulations), and may be prevented or treated with atropine. Atrial premature contractions (APCs) are commonly caused by stimulation under too light anaesthesia (particularly dental extraction). In the latter case, treatment with a beta blocker may be necessary.

(2) Ventricular dysrhythmias occur for a variety of reasons. Dental extraction is a common cause of multi-focal ectopics occurring in the otherwise normal patient. In rare circumstances this may lead to ventricular tachycardia or even fibrillation. Again, treatment with beta blockers or lignocaine usually reduces their frequency and severity. If the sinus rate slows excessively (see above), 'opportunist' ectopics may occur, but these are usually easily overridden by simply increasing the heart rate with atropine. A common accompaniment of halothane anaesthesia is ventricular bigeminus, particularly if there is an element of CO_2 retention during spontaneous respiration (Fig. 4.13b). This is not usually serious, but can be alleviated by reduction of halothane concentration and/or lowering the $PaCO_2$ by ventilatory assistance for a short period. In more resistant cases, halothane may have to be discontinued and substituted by other inhalational agents less likely to cause dysrhythmias such as enflurane and isoflurane.

The concurrent administration of adrenaline (during local anaesthetic infiltration) may precipitate serious ventricular dysrhythmias in association with high concentrations of halothane and CO_2 retention. This should not occur if the dose of adrenaline is limited to about $0.15 \, \text{ml} \, \text{kg}^{-1}$ of a $1:100\,000$ mixture $(10 \, \mu\text{g} \, \text{ml}^{-1})$ over a 10 minute period, and hypoxia and hypercarbia are avoided.

(d) Ischaemia detection

During anaesthesia, the principal method of ischaemia detection involves the ST segment. Provided the machine is correctly calibrated (1 mV for 1 cm upward deflection) and the filters switched off, ST segment depression of more than 1 mm signifies impending subendocardial ischaemia. This usually indicates that the oxygen supply/demand ratio of the heart has been adversely affected, e.g. oxygen demand is excessive, as in tachycardia and hypertension in the patient with pre-existing ischaemic myocardium, or supply is reduced as in excessive hypotension (Chapter 14). Correction of these factors should return the ST segment to normality. ST segment elevation is less common, but may signify full thickness myocardial ischaemia with impending infarction. If possible surgery should be completed expeditiously and anaesthesia discontinued, as it is extremely likely to lead to 'full blown' myocardial infarction.

(e) Conclusion

Even in the 'normal' patient, ECG monitoring gives extremely useful information which can be appropriately acted upon with benefit to the patient, as indicated above. Two things should be noted with caution, first, a normal ECG has no absolute correlation with blood pressure and perfusion, it simply reflects the electrical (and not mechanical) activity of the heart. Secondly, the biggest changes in cardiovascular homeostasis usually occur when the ECG is not being monitored (in the UK at least), i.e. during induction and intubation.

5
Anaesthetic drugs

Those unfamiliar with basic pharmacological principles (e.g. pharmacokinetics, pharmacodynamics) should refer to Appendix A. Pharmacokinetic data for many of the drugs referred to in this chapter is available on page 130.

Anaesthetic Gases and Vapours

Introduction

The administration of anaesthetic gases and volatile agents to render the patient unconscious is one of the few therapeutic interventions in medicine which involve the lung as the portal of entry to the body to produce a systemic effect. The reasons behind this are mainly historical, but the continuing lack of suitable intravenous anaesthetics to produce an equivalent state means that this mode of administration will continue for the forseeable future. Indeed, the rapid elimination through the airway is probably the most important factor for their popularity.

Definition

Inhaled agents which produce unconsciousness are many and varied, but in anaesthesia they can be divided into two main groups:

(a) The anaesthetic gases, nitrous oxide and cyclopropane: these agents are gaseous at room temperature and pressure, but may be liquefied under pressure, i.e. their critical temperature is above room temperature.

(Critical temperature is the temperature of a gas above which it may not be liquefied whatever the applied pressure.)

(b) The volatile agents, halothane, enflurane and isoflurane: these agents are liquids at room temperature and pressure, but they are volatile and vaporise easily (i.e. their boiling point is low, approximately 50–60°C).

Mode of Action

The precise way in which these agents work is still hotly debated, but certain facts can be stated. Parts of the central nervous system are intimately associated with preservation of consciousness, such as the reticular activating system in the mid brain. Surgical ablation of this area produces irreversible coma in animals, whereas anaesthetic gases and volatile agents can produce reversible coma by obtunding synaptic transmission. This ability is thought to be due, in part, to the lipophilic nature of these agents, whereby they modify the lipid constituents in the synaptic cell membrane and thus block ionic events (such as in the sodium channel) which are necessary for cell to cell transmission. When administration of the agent is discontinued, synaptic transmission is restored and the patient awakens. General anaesthetics do not seem to act by binding to specific receptors. An interesting and scientifically important phenomenon is that the anaesthetic effect of volatile agents can be reversed by subjecting the whole animal to high ambient pressures (50–100 atmospheres). This indicates that the interaction of the agent with the cell membrane may be of a 'physical' nature, perhaps by modifying the geometry of the bilipid layer or its interaction with protein constituents.

Principles of Administration of Anaesthetic Gases and Volatile Agents

To ensure that the mixture of carrier gas and vapour reaches the patient in a similar concentration to that leaving the vaporiser and flow meters, non-rebreathing systems are employed. This is not true, however, with systems utilising low 'fresh gas' flows, carbon dioxide absorption and rebreathing of expired gas. The difficulty in accurately predicting the inspired tension of inhaled vapours with such systems has resulted in them being less popular, especially amongst inexperienced anaesthetists.

(a) Minimum alveolar concentration (MAC)

The concentration of agents that are necessary to produce and safely to maintain unconsciousness must be known. This has been greatly facilitated by the concept of 'MAC', which is the alveolar concentration of the agent which will prevent movement to a reproducible surgical stimulus in 50% of subjects. Several points emerge, first MAC is not the inspired concentration (i.e. that set on the flowmeters and vaporiser), but the concentration in the alveoli after the anaesthetic agents have mixed with the alveolar gases, oxygen, nitrogen and so on. During induction of anaesthesia, the inspired tension of inhaled vapour is much greater than expired (alveolar) but becomes roughly equilibrated (depending on the solubility of the agent in blood) after about 20 minutes or so. Secondly, as MAC refers to only 50% of subjects, the concept of 'AD$_{95}$' has been put forward to include 95%, and is roughly 1.5 times the MAC concentration.

(b) Principles of induction and maintenance

As has been seen, unconsciousness is produced in the central nervous system, but MAC (or

AD$_{95}$) refers to alveoli. In fact, the decrease in tension (partial pressure) of the anaesthetic gas or volatile agent is minimal between the alveoli and the brain. What is necessary, is to produce a rapid rise in alveolar anaesthetic tension to the level of 1.5 × MAC, maintain it during the operation, and stop administration to allow the patient to awaken at the end of the procedure. The following factors increase the rate of rise of alveolar anaesthetic tension as a fraction of inspired values (i.e. FA/FI).

(1) Increased minute volume of ventilation
(2) Increased concentration of the gas or vapour
(3) Decreased cardiac output
(4) Decreased blood/gas solubility
(5) Increased venous anaesthetic tension

(1) and (2) increase delivery of agent to the alveoli, (3), (4) and (5) decrease the rate at which the blood passing through the lungs removes the agent, which would otherwise tend to lower alveolar concentration (remember it is the partial pressure of the agent in the alveoli and blood, not the physical amount, which determines the degree of unconsciousness). Just as it is necessary to give a bolus of an intravenous drug to achieve a desired level, and an infusion to maintain it, so in this case an inhalational bolus is given (the concentration being higher initially than the expected maintenance) followed by the maintenance level.

The Stages of Anaesthesia

MAC levels can only be a rough guide to the amount of agent required, due to individual variation, and thus the anaesthetist must be aware of the response of each patient as depth of anaesthesia varies. Guedel devised a classification for ether anaesthesia which has remained a classic description of the progression from the awake to the deeply anaesthetised state. It is rarely seen in modern anaesthesia, since it only applies to inhalational induction; the progression is too rapid with intravenous agents.

(a) Stage 1: Induction

This stage lasts from the moment that administration begins until the patient no longer responds to questions. With some agents, e.g. ether and nitrous oxide, significant analgesia is present during this stage and this fact is utilised for pain relief in labour with inhalation of nitrous oxide 50% with oxygen ('Entonox').

(b) Stage 2: Excitement

There follows a period of hyperreflexia which is prolonged with ether, short with halothane, during which the patient may struggle, cough, incur bronchospasm, vomit and so on. Pupils are dilated and respiration irregular.

(c) Stage 3: Surgical anaesthesia

This is divided into 4 planes during which the patient becomes progressively more deeply anaesthetised, with regular respiration and no response to stimuli. Pupils are small in plane 1, and increase progressively in diameter towards plane 4. Plane 2 is adequate for peripheral operations, or major surgery combined with neuromuscular blockers. If full relaxation has to be achieved with a purely inhalational technique, plane 3 or even 4 must be reached. It must be emphasised that Plane 4 is perilously close to medullary paralysis and cardiac arrest (Stage 4).

(d) Stage 4: Medullary paralysis

This stage should never be reached. The patient is apnoeic with profound respiratory and cardiovascular depression. Cardiac arrest quickly ensues unless the concentration of the agent is quickly reduced and oxygenation and normocapnoea restored.

The Place of Inhalational Anaesthesia

In recent years it has become increasingly appreciated that high flows of anaesthetic gases and vapours which emanate from the expiratory valves of anaesthetic breathing systems may have serious adverse effects on theatre personnel. This pollution has spurred on the development of purely intravenous techniques to

obviate this problem, but lack of suitable agents has meant that this has not received wide acceptance. Instead, costly anti-pollution systems have been used to duct the offending gases away from the theatre environment, although a simpler approach would be to employ low flow closed circuit techniques. Thus, virtually all anaesthetics will consist of at least nitrous oxide and often small quantities of an inhalational agent such as halothane. The rationale for the various combinations used is discussed in Chapter 1.

The doses and actions of commonly used inhalational agents are given in Table 5.1

Intravenous Anaesthetics

Definition and Mode of Action

Intravenous anaesthetics produce general anaesthesia when given in appropriate doses. There is loss of consciousness and insensibility to surgical stimuli, with cardiovascular and respiratory depression dependent upon the drug and dose used. Their action is short (5–15 minutes) following a single dose.

Large doses of analgesics, e.g. morphine, or sedatives, e.g. diazepam, may also produce unconsciousness but otherwise do not fall within the definition.

The mode of action of intravenous anaesthetics is thought to be similar to that of inhalational agents.

Principles of Administration

(a) As these agents are administered intravenously, patient co-operation is only required during venous access, although this may be difficult in the uncooperative, very young or obese patient. Gaseous induction of anaesthesia, on the other hand, is often punctuated by breath holding, excessive secretions, laryngospasm and so on which makes the process both difficult and protracted.

(b) With inhalational agents, anaesthesia progresses through stages over the course of several

TABLE 5.1 **Doses and actions of some commonly used inhalational agents**

Agent	% concentration at 1.5 MAC with 60% N₂O	Time to equilibration (min)	Respiration	Blood pressure	Side effects	Analgesic effects
Halothane	1	20	depressed	down	hypotension, bradycardia, hepatic failure	No
Enflurane	2.4	15	depressed	down	hypotension	No
Isoflurane	1.8	15	depressed	down	hypotension	No
Tricholorethylene	0.2	40	tachypnoea	—	dysrhythmias, cannot be used with soda lime†	Yes
Nitrous oxide	*	5	—	—	not potent	Yes

* The MAC of nitrous oxide is 103%, so it is impossible, at atmospheric pressure, to give MAC values without incurring hypoxia.
† The exposure of soda lime to trichloroethylene results in the formation of toxic 'nerve gases' such as phosgene.

minutes, the process being reversible by simply switching off the vaporiser and allowing the anaesthetic to be eliminated via the airway. With intravenous anaesthetics, once in the patient, recovery is dependent upon redistribution and metabolism within the body.

(c) Once in the blood stream, the agent needs to reach the brain in sufficient concentration to affect synaptic transmission within the reticular activating system (presumed main site of action). All other tissues in the body receive their share of drug depending on regional blood flow.

The ideal induction agent should have a highly specific action within the brain; unfortunately, all other excitable tissues will be affected in a dose-dependent manner. Nearly all the induction agents depress the myocardium directly. In patients with severe cardiac disease there is a narrow margin between the dose of anaesthetic causing unconsciousness and that causing excessive cardiac depression.

Another instance where great care must be exercised in the administration of an intravenous anaesthetic is in severe dehydration and

hypovolaemia; in these situations blood pressure is maintained by a high level of central sympathetic activity; the usual dose of intravenous agent can have diastrous effects by reducing central sympathetic drive and simultaneously depressing the heart. Fluid repletion is obviously necessary before surgery and anaesthesia.

(d) Drugs are distributed within the body following different patterns (Appendix A). Thiopentone, the most popular induction agent, is often given as an example of a drug possessing short action by virtue of redistribution. When given as a single bolus, its effect within the brain is short, but the drug remains as an active compound within other tissues of the body, being only slowly metabolised in the liver ('hangover effect'). Some of the breakdown products are also active and are eliminated by the kidney. Up to 48 hours are needed for complete elimination, and within that time the effects of other sedative drugs or alcohol are potentiated.

(e) For day case surgery thiopentone is often avoided for the reasons given above. Other intravenous agents are usually preferred such as methohexitone and etomidate. The latter is rapidly metabolised in the liver into inactive compounds.

(f) Anaesthesia may be maintained by infusion of intravenous anaesthetics. However, at present, there is only one potentially suitable drug available which combines safety with short duration of action. As a result, this technique has had limited popularity, although the implications for reduction of pollution are obvious.

Choice of Induction Agent

There are five induction agents in current use in the UK (Table 5.2). The ideal agent is still a long way in the future; thiopentone continues to occupy a prominent place in this group of drugs.

Neuromuscular Blockade

Definition

A neuromuscular blocking drug (NMB) is one which specifically prevents the passage of an impulse from nerve to muscle. In doing so, muscular relaxation is achieved, thus allowing operations to be carried out intra-abdominally or intrathoracically which would otherwise require excessive amounts of inhalational anaesthetics.

Mode of Action

In abdominal surgery, skin incision or handling of the gut leads to contraction of the abdominal muscles as a protective reflex. In a similar

TABLE 5.2   Summary of induction agents

Agent	Chemical group	Dose (mg/70 kg fit man)	Cessation of action (min)	CVS	Pain on injection	Other effects
Thiopentone (Intraval, Pentothal)	barbiturate	500	10 redistribution	depression	rare	hangover, cumul eff
Methohexitone (Brietal)	barbiturate	100	8 redistribution	depression	++	invol mov, cumul eff
Etomidate (Hypnomidate)	imidazole derivative	20	8 liver metabolism	minimal depression	+++	invol mov, nausea, suppression of cortical hormones
Propofol (~~Ativan~~) (Diprivan)	phenol derivative	150	8 liver metabolism	depression	++	respiratory depression
Ketamine (Ketalar)	phencyclidine derivative	150	15 liver metabolism	stimulation	none	hallucinations analgesia

Key: CVS   – effects upon the cardiovascular system.
    hallucinations – occurring during the recovery phase
    invol mov   – involuntary movement appearing after induction
    cumul eff   – cumulative effect, i.e. rapid redistribution, but slow elimination phase
    liver metabolism– fall in plasma levels due to inactivation of drug in liver
    redistribution   – fall in plasma levels due to redistribution of the drug to less well-perfused tissues

fashion, the same muscles will contract if one is punched in the stomach. To abolish this response with non-specific depressants, such as halothane, would require doses much in excess of that necessary for unconsciousness, and this may lead to depression of vital organs apart from the brain, such as the heart and liver. The chemical transmitter at the neuromuscular junction is acetylcholine (ACh) and following its release, it binds reversibly to receptors on the muscle side, producing depolarisation and contraction. A NMB specifically interrupts this process, thus paralysing the muscle and obviating the need for high doses of central depressants. NMBs are of two types:

(a) Depolarisers

Examples are suxamethonium and decamethonium. They bind to the ACh receptor but cause a more prolonged depolarisation than ACh, the muscle being unexcitable and insensitive to ACh. Initial, uncoordinated, contractions are seen followed by paralysis which lasts about 5 minutes with suxamethonium and 20 minutes with decamethonium.

It should be noted that NMBs are highly ionised compounds and do not cross the blood–brain barrier, so they exert no central depressant effects. This fact must be borne in mind when prescribing them to 'settle' patients who require artificial ventilation in the intensive care unit. Concomitant administration of a sedative is mandatory.

(b) Competitive

Tubocurarine, gallamine, alcuronium, pancuronium, atracurium and vecuronium are competitive antagonists of ACh, i.e. they prevent ACh activating specific receptors on the postsynaptic membrane, thus producing paralysis.

Termination of Action of Neuromuscular blockers

(a) Depolarisers

The normal action of ACh at the neuromuscular junction is terminated by the enzyme acetylcholinesterase (AChE) which breaks it down in less than one millisecond, thus allowing the active site to repolarise and further muscular contraction to take place. Suxamethonium is metabolised by a naturally occurring esterase, pseudocholinesterase (PsChE), which is found in plasma and tissues. Although similar to AChE, it acts more slowly, thus accounting for the 5 minute duration of suxamethonium. Some people have a defective PsChE which means that the action of suxamethonium is considerably prolonged ('Suxamethonium apnoea').

Decamethonium relies entirely on renal excretion, with a duration of 15 to 20 minutes.

(b) Competitive

It may be several hours before complete recovery of neuromuscular function occurs following a standard dose of tubocurarine or pancuronium. A reversal agent is usually employed to hasten this process. As these agents work by competition with ACh, the concentration of the latter may be increased by inhibiting AChE with an anti-AChE such as neostigmine. Provided some recovery of neuromuscular transmission has occurred, the extra ACh will overcome the residual effect of the block and 'normal' function will be restored. Being a non-specific anti-AChE, neostigmine causes accumulation of ACh at muscarinic as well as nicotinic sites (Appendix B). This leads to vagal effects such as bradycardia, bronchospasm, increased gut motility and so on. The muscarinic effects should be simultaneously blocked by atropine, which, although being a competitive blocker of ACh (like tubocurarine), has no effect on the neuromuscular junction. The standard dose for a 70 kg adult is neostigmine 2.5 mg and atropine 1.2 mg.

The newer NMBs such as atracurium and vecuronium have a much faster recovery than earlier drugs and in some instances reverse spontaneously, or at the very least require lower doses of neostigmine to restore neuromuscular function.

Clinical Uses

(a) Intubation of the trachea. Suxamethonium is often employed as it produces rapid, profound and short-lived paralysis. This allows intubation under light anaesthesia, and is especially useful if this is necessary to protect the airway from aspiration of gastric contents during emergency surgery (Chapter 8).

(b) To produce muscular relaxation for abdominal or thoracic surgery which would otherwise require regional techniques or very deep inhalational anaesthesia.

(c) To assist in the control of ventilation, e.g. intensive care unit (Chapter 10).

(d) To prevent reflex muscle activity during light anaesthesia.

(e) To control muscle spasm, e.g. tetanus and electroconvulsive therapy (ECT).

Monitoring Neuromuscular Transmission

During operations in which competitive NMBs are employed, neuromuscular transmission should be monitored by a peripheral nerve stimulator (PNS) as it is impossible to be sure of the contribution of anaesthesia itself to 'relaxation'. Similarly, at the end of the procedure, neuromuscular transmission must be fully restored with appropriate doses of neostigmine and atropine and checking that this is so with a PNS, before a clinical assessment of adequacy of reversal is made. The latter includes head raising, squeezing the hand, ability to cough, and so on. It is absolutely essential that the patient has complete recovery of neuromuscular transmission before recovering consciousness.

Choice of Neuromuscular Blocker

This is referred to in Table 5.3. Generally speaking, where intubation is necessary but spontaneous respiration is planned, suxamethonium is used. If the operation is of longer duration and requires profound muscular relaxation, a competitive blocker is employed, and this may

TABLE 5.3   Characteristics of neuromuscular blockers

Neuromuscular blocker	Dose $(mg\ kg^{-1})$	Duration (min)	Blood pressure	Side effects	Contra-indications
Suxamethonium (Scoline, Anectine)	1 to 2	5–10	up	muscle pains, bradycardia, increase in plasma K^+	absent PsChE, hyperkalaemia, open eye injury, myotonias, paraplegia, burns
Tubocurarine (Jexin, Tubarine)	0.5	45	down	hypotension, histamine release	myasthenia, shock
Gallamine (Flaxedil)	2.0	35	up	tachycardia	renal failure
Alcuronium (Alloferin)	0.25	35	down	histamine release	myasthenia
Pancuronium (Pavulon)	0.08	40	up	hypertension	myasthenia
Atracurium (Tracrium)	0.5	25	—	histamine release if dose >0.8 mg kg^{-1}	—
Vecuronium (Norcuron)	0.08	25	—	—	—

also be used to facilitate intubation. For short operations with intermittent positive pressure ventilation, one of the more rapidly acting agents such as atracurium or vecuronium will confer advantages. If the patient is shocked pancuronium, which facilitates sympathetic transmission, is preferable to tubocurarine which blocks it.

Myasthenia gravis is a contra-indication for the use of competitive NMBs because of prolonged paralysis. Vecuronium and atracurium are probably suitable, in small doses.

Chronic respiratory disease is also a relative contra-indication for the use of competitive NMBs, because the fatigued respiratory muscles are more susceptible to the drugs.

Local Anaesthetic Drugs

Of all anaesthetic agents, local anaesthetics are perhaps those most widely used by non-anaesthetists. Serious and fatal complications associated with their use have escalated in recent years.

Lignocaine

Pharmacological properties

Lignocaine is the most frequently used drug in this group. It may be used as a local anaesthetic, as an anti-dysrhythmic or as a general anaesthetic.

(1) As a local anaesthetic agent, lignocaine may be used as a 4% cream, or fluid for topical application, as a 2% solution for nerve blocks. 1.5% for epidurals, 0.5–1% for local infiltration of tissues, and as 0.5% for intravenous regional anaesthesia (Bier's block). With the exception of the intravenous, epidural and topical application, it is usually given mixed with adrenaline in the strength of $1:200000$ or $5\,\mu g$ in $1\,ml$. Adrenaline significantly reduces the absorption of lignocaine from tissues, therefore delaying uptake and prolonging its local effect.

As a local anaesthetic, the total amount administered over one hour must not exceed a maximum of 250 mg in the fit average 70 kg adult, when given as a plain solution. With adrenaline, the maximum dose can be increased to 500 mg ($3\,mg\,kg^{-1}$, plain and $6\,mg\,kg^{-1}$ with adrenaline). Proportionately smaller maximum doses apply to smaller body weight, and great caution should be exercised with its use in the elderly and the very ill.

Duration of action depends on the type of block and on the total amount given. It averages approximately 1 hour for plain lignocaine and 2–3 hours if used with adrenaline.

(2) As an anti-dysrhythmic agent, lignocaine is given intravenously as a 1–2% solution. It is indicated in the treatment of ventricular dysrhythmias. Initially, $1.5\,mg\,kg^{-1}$ can be given as a bolus injection, followed by half this amount 10 minutes later if necessary. If effective, a continuous intravenous infusion (0.8%, 4 g in 500 ml) may be set up at a starting rate of $30\,\mu g\,kg^{-1}\,min^{-1}$ ($2\,mg\,min^{-1}$ in a 70 kg patient). A maximum rate of $50\,\mu g\,kg^{-1}\,min^{-1}$ should not be exceeded because of the likelihood of inducing general anaesthesia followed by cardiac and respiratory depression.

(3) As a general anaesthetic, lignocaine can be used at a rate of $100\,\mu g\,kg^{-1}\,min^{-1}$ intravenously. Because of its general analgesic effects it may be used instead of a narcotic analgesic, supplemented with nitrous oxide, in balanced anaesthesia. This technique is often favoured for surgery of the middle ear, especially if labyrinthine symptoms are present, since the latter are usually aggravated by narcotic analgesics.

Pharmcokinetics

The distribution and elimination of lignocaine is probably one of the best studied. The half-life of the redistribution phase is approximately 10 minutes, but the half-life of the slower elimination phase is nearly 2 hours.

Side effects

The main side effects of lignocaine are due to an exaggeration of its therapeutic effects upon excitable tissues, namely depression of the central nervous system and of the conductive tissue of the heart, as outlined above. Depression of the central nervous system may be preceded by excitation.

The first sign of overdosage in the awake patient is usually the sensation of tingling in the tongue and lips. Shortly afterwards the patient looks pale, and feels anxious and nauseated. Unconsciousness may soon follow, or may be preceded by an epileptiform convulsion. At this point the full skills of a trained anaesthetist are required. The patient may have a very low blood pressure and respiratory depression; full resuscitation measures are needed.

Bupivacaine (Marcaine)

Bupivacaine is second to lignocaine in frequency of use. It is about four times more potent and four times more toxic than lignocaine. The duration of action is much longer, and for this reason it is often preferred; in nerve blocks its effects normally last 4–6 hours.

Bupivacaine is used for epidural analgesia in obstetrics for two additional reasons: first, it crosses the placental barrier at a much slower rate, reaching the fetus in lesser amounts; and secondly, it causes a smaller degree of motor paralysis than lignocaine or any other local anaesthetic agent for the same amount of sensory blockade. This is an important advantage in analgesia for vaginal delivery.

It is used as 0.25%, 0.5% or 0.75% plain solutions. In labour, the 0.25% solution or an intermediate 0.375% are used initially. The 0.75% solution has been recently introduced and its advantages over the 0.5% solution are yet to be established. Indeed recent experience suggests that the 0.75% solution may be more toxic.

The side effects of bupivacaine are similar to those of lignocaine; the occurrence of convulsions due to overdosage has been claimed to be more frequent.

Prilocaine (Citanest)

Prilocaine is only slightly less potent than lignocaine, but much less toxic (higher therapeutic index as a local anaesthetic). It has a duration of action in between lignocaine and bupivacaine. In high doses (more than 600 mg) it may cause methaemoglobinaemia. Because of its low toxicity, prilocaine is recommended for intravenous regional anaesthesia in the strength of 0.5%; volumes up to 40 ml can be safely used in the average fit adult. It is also of value as a surface anaesthetic, in 2% solution, for fibre-optic bronchoscopy in the awake patient.

Other Local Anaesthetic Agents

The following are much less frequently used:

(a) Cocaine in topical anaesthesia of the nasal mucosa and conjunctiva; it has a marked vasoconstrictor effect.
(b) Procaine is rarely used due to its short duration of action (metabolised by plasma pseudocholinesterase).
(c) Amethocaine, mostly used as a topical analgesic in the UK and as a spinal analgesic in the US.
(d) Cinchocaine (Nupercaine, Dibucaine) is used for spinal anaesthesia as a 'heavy solution' in 5% dextrose, and in the *in vitro* test for plasma pseudocholinesterase activity ('Dibucaine number').
(e) Mepivacaine (Carbocaine) also used for spinals and epidurals.
(f) Etidocaine is used in epidural analgesia.

NB. The concentration of local anaesthetics is often given as '% solution'. To avoid toxicity it is necessary to limit the dose of these agents on a $mg\,kg^{-1}$ basis. 1% (1 in 100) solution means that there is 1 g of the substance in 100 ml or 10 mg per ml. Thus, 10 ml of 1% lignocaine = 100 mg. A concentration of solution less than 1% is often expressed as, for example, 1 in 1000, 1 in 10 000 and so on. 1 in 1000 is 1 g in 1000 ml or $1\,mg\,ml^{-1}$, 1 in 10 000 is 1 g in 10 000 ml or 1 mg in 10 ml.

Analgesics; Post-operative Pain; Antiemetics

Definition and Types of Analgesics

Analgesics are substances which raise the pain threshold. They may be divided into 4 main groups, the non-steroidal anti-inflammatory drugs, the opiate agonists, the opiate agonist–antagonists and partial agonists, and miscellaneous drugs whose site of action is unknown. It should be remembered that these drugs, as a rule, do not attempt to cure the condition causing the pain, but are purely symptomatic, e.g. following surgery, where natural healing processes eventually remove the cause of pain. Other drugs may produce analgesia by actually removing the pain causing condition, e.g. nitrates in angina, carbamazepine in trigeminal neuralgia and ergot in migraine.

(a) Non-steroidal anti-inflammatory drugs (NSAIDs)

These include aspirin, paracetamol (although not anti-inflammatory), and the newer drugs such as ibuprofen and piroxicam. Their primary use post-operatively is for pain relief once it has subsided to the point where opiates are no longer necessary, usually when the patient begins to ambulate. They may have a useful additive action with opiates, and are often used concurrently. Other uses are for treatment of pyrexia in the intensive care unit (ICU, Chapter 15) and in cancer pain, particularly if there is bony involvement (Chapter 17).

Paracetamol is the drug of choice as it does not have the side effects of other drugs in this group, e.g. gastric irritation and bleeding or platelet dysfunction. It is given in a dose of two tablets (1 g) 6 hourly.

(b) Opiate agonists

These include morphine, pethidine, papaveretum (a mixture of opiate alkaloids) and the intra-operative analgesics fentanyl, alfentanil and phenoperidine.

Actions

They work both spinally and in areas of the brain stem rich in naturally occurring opioid peptides, such as the periaqueductal and periventricular grey matter (Chapter 17). Beneficial actions, apart from analgesia, include euphoria and anxiolysis. Side effects are common and can have serious consequences, such as nausea and vomiting, respiratory depression, constipation, urinary retention, sedation, itching, tachyphylaxis and addiction.

Administration

They are usually administered intramuscularly (Table 5.4). The standard post-operative prescription has been shown to result in a tenfold variation in plasma levels of the drug, in similar-sized patients. This means that the dosage must be individualised. In ambulant or post-operative patients they may also be given orally, but the majority undergo significant 'first pass' metabolism in the liver; with morphine the oral dose must be five times higher than the intramuscular dose. First pass metabolism is highly dependent on liver blood flow and should this be reduced, as following blood loss, the effectiveness of the drug is enhanced leading to toxicity. Intravenous administration produces more reliable and immediate drug levels and effects, but is usually restricted to high dependency areas (with higher nurse:patient ratios than are found on general wards) due to the danger of respiratory depression. Patient-controlled analgesia (PCA) apparatus for post-

TABLE 5.4 Doses of opiate agonists used (70 kg patient)

	Intramuscularly	*Orally*	*Frequency*
Morphine	10–15 mg	30 mg	4 hourly
Pethidine	75–100 mg	50–150 mg	3 hourly
Papaveretum	15–20 mg	20 mg	4 hourly

operative use is becoming more common, and may be safely set up on general wards.

Uses

As they are addictive, their uses is restricted to severe pain, such as post-operative, myocardial infarction, renal colic and cancer. Their euphoric side effects make them useful premedicants, and, together with the tendency to depress respiration, have led to their use in ICU for sedating patients undergoing mechanical ventilation.

(c) Opiate agonist–antagonists and partial agonists

Actions

The side effects of conventional opiate agonists led to the development of a new class of compound, the antagonist analgesics. They were so called because they originated from the morphine antagonist nalorphine, which was only later discovered to have analgesic properties of its own. Because of its unfortunate propensity to cause dysphoria it is not clinically useful as an analgesic, but it does not seem to produce as serious respiratory depression or addiction as the conventional opiates such as morphine. It led to the development of more clinically useful compounds such as pentazocine and nalbuphine.

Their ability to antagonise opiate agonists, and yet have analgesic properties of their own has led to the proposition of three different types of opiate receptors, named 'mu', 'kappa' and 'sigma'. Conventional opiates are agonists and produce analgesia at the mu (named after mor-phine) receptor at which pentazocine and nalbuphine are antagonists. The latter produce analgesia at the kappa (keto-cyclazocine) receptor and dysphoria at the sigma (SKF drug, nor-metazocine) receptor. This would explain why nalorphine is unable to antagonise the respiratory depression of pentazocine, but naloxone (a pure mu and kappa antagonist) is. Side effects include dysphoria, nausea and vomiting (pentazocine more than nalbuphine) and respiratory depression. They are not as efficacious as the opiate agonists.

Buprenorphine is a partial agonist derived from thebaine, an opiate alkaloid. It produces analgesia at the mu receptor but exhibits a ceiling of activity for respiratory depression and possibly for analgesia. If given after low doses of opiate agonists it has an additive analgesic action, whereas following a large dose it may be antagonistic. Its great avidity for the receptor accounts for its long duration of action, its low abuse potential, and difficulty in reversal with naloxone. It does not cause dysphoria, but respiratory depression is enhanced by sedative drugs such as diazepam.

Dose

The doses used are given in Table 5.5.

Uses

These are similar to the opiate agonists. However, pentazocine is not recommended for myocardial infarction as it tends to increase right heart work. The alternating use of the opiate agonists and the agonist–antagonists is to be deprecated.

TABLE 5.5   Doses of opiate agonist–antagonists used (70 kg patient)

	Intramuscularly	Orally	Frequency
Pentazocine	30–60 mg	50–100 mg	3 hourly
Nalbuphine	10–20 mg		3 hourly
Buprenorphine	0.3–0.6 mg	0.4–0.6 mg (sublingually)	6 hourly

Miscellaneous

Nefopam and meptazinol are unique strong analgesics whose site of action is less clear than with the other opiates, but there appears to be a reduced tendency to produce respiratory depression. Other side effects are unpredictable.

Ketamine is a powerful analgesic in subanaesthetic doses of 20–40 mg; it causes sympathetic stimulation and marked hallucinations (probably via the sigma receptor) which can be attenuated with diazepam.

Post-operative Analgesia

Although surgery is classically categorised into minor, intermediate and major, the perception of pain does not recognise these artificial boundaries, and some patients will experience considerably more pain following inguinal hernia repair, which is an intermediate operation, than others following cholecystecomy, a major operation. Analgesic drugs are prescribed by doctors but administered by nurses who may have unfounded fears concerning addiction with opiates. Respiratory depression is certainly possible and may be potentiated by depressant drugs given during anaesthesia. Due to these fears, analgesics are often withheld from patients who are nevertheless in pain. It is thus understandable that self-administration apparatus and longer-acting analgesics may become more popular.

Doses

These are as outlined in the section on analgesics, but it must be emphasised that the dose and administration interval should be tailored to suit the individual patient.

Other methods of analgesia

These include regional techniques such as epidural analgesia (with bupivacaine or opiates), paravertebral or intercostal nerve block, or even simple infiltration of the wound with a local anaesthetic (Chapter 18). Transcutaneous nerve stimulation, acupuncture and hypnosis are only successful in a small percentage of patients.

Antiemetics

(a) Pathways of nausea and vomiting

The two structures intimately involved are the chemoreceptor trigger zone (CTZ) and the emetic centre (EC), both found in the medulla close to the vital centres around the floor of the fourth ventricle. The CTZ is outside the blood–brain barrier. The EC may be stimulated directly by impulses arising in the labyrinth (vertigo, motion sickness), meninges (raised intracranial pressure), cortex (psychogenic) or the periphery (gastrointestinal tract). It may also be stimulated by impulses arising from the CTZ. The transmitters involved at the EC appear to be histamine (H1 receptor) and acetylcholine. The CTZ is stimulated by drugs such as opiates and digoxin, metabolic causes such as uraemia, pregnancy hormones and cytotoxics. The transmitter involved here is dopamine. This provides for rational treatment of vomiting according to the anticipated causation: dopamine antagonists are effective for opiates but not for travel sickness where the antihistamines would be more suitable. The proximity of the CTZ to the area of highest density of opiate receptors should be noted.

Apart from drugs, it should also be remembered that the site of surgery is important; gynaecological operations, particularly, are very prone to cause unpleasant nausea and vomiting in the immediate post-operative period.

Patients should be reassured pre-operatively that, should they suffer nausea and vomiting, specific drugs are available and are administered on demand.

(b) Drug groups

(1) *Antihistamines*
These work at the EC and are particularly useful in travel sickness, e.g. cyclizine 50 mg orally or 25–50 mg intravenously. This may be combined with morphine for post-operative use as an i.m. preparation. Side effects include sedation and possible allergic reactions.

(2) *Anticholinergics*
These work at the EC also, e.g. hyoscine 0.2–

TABLE 5.6   Dopamine antagonist antiemetics

	Example	Intramuscular dose	Frequency
Phenothiazines	perphenazine	2.5–5 mg	4 hourly
Butyrophenones	droperidol	2.5–5 mg	6 hourly
Procainamide derivatives	metoclopramide	10–20 mg	8 hourly
Benzimidazole derivatives	domperidone	10–20 mg	6 hourly

0.6 mg intramuscularly or orally, and may be combined with papaveretum for premedication.

(3) *Dopamine antagonists*

These are made up of 4 main groups (Table 5.6). They work primarily at the CTZ having less effect on those stimuli producing nausea and vomiting at the EC. They are useful to counteract the nausea and vomiting which result from the administration of opiate drugs. The phenothiazines include some which are also antihistamines and anticholinergics, such as promethazine, so they have additional activity at the emetic centre. Together with the butyrophenones they are also major tranquillisers.

The central antidopaminergic action of all these drugs may precipitate Parkinsonism in susceptible patients. If the recommended dose is exceeded in normal individuals a serious, occasionally fatal, extrapyramidal syndrome may develop. Domperidone is claimed to be devoid of such side effects.

Metoclopramide and domperidone increase intestinal motility and gastric emptying.

Note: All doses referred to are for a 70 kg healthy patient. For other body weights and more susceptible patients suitable adjustments can be made. Generally speaking, dividing the adult dose (mentioned in the text) by 70 gives a $mg\,kg^{-1}$ figure which is suitable for the majority of patients. At the extremes of age (e.g. <1 year and the elderly) half the calculated dose should be administered initially and scaled up or down as appropriate. In shocked patients (e.g. following trauma or major burns) a much smaller dose is administered i.v. (e.g. 2.5 mg papaveretum per 70 kg) as tissue perfusion and patient response is very variable in this situation.

6

Peri-operative fluid management; blood and colloid administration; coagulation disorders

Water and Electrolyte Balance

This section is concerned with the fluid and electrolyte requirements of the short period of time immediately preceding and following uneventful surgery (48 to 72 hours). Only water, sodium and potassium will be considered. Requirements for longer-term therapy should be considered in the context of total intravenous feeding (Chapter 15). Blood loss and replacement is discussed later and losses arising from burns are dealt with in Chapter 16.

Body Contents

Approximate contents of the body in water, Na and K of a 70 kg body weight adult male:

Total body water: 40 litres or 60% of b.w. (52% in female).

Total body sodium: 4000 mmol or 55 mmol kg^{-1} b.w.

Total body potassium: 3000 mmol or 45 mmol kg^{-1} b.w.

Daily Requirements

Normal daily requirements of a 70 kg adult:

Water: 2.5 litres (use paediatric table for less than 60 kg)
Na$^+$: 100 mmol or 1.5 mmol kg^{-1} b.w.
K$^+$: 70 mmol or 1 mmol kg^{-1} b.w.

Paediatric Values

Paediatric requirements for water are based on body surface area rather than weight. A useful rule based upon body weight is as follows:

kg body weight	ml kg^{-1} 24 h^{-1}	ml kg^{-1} h^{-1}
First 10	100	4
Next 10	50	2
Remaining	20	1

Example:
A 35 kg child will need daily

	1000 ml water	(10 kg @ 100)
+	500 ml	(10 kg @ 50)
+	300 ml	(15 kg @ 20)

Total 1800 ml

Intravenous Fluids

The composition of commonly used intravenous fluids is given in Table 6.1.

TABLE 6.1. Composition of intravenous fluids (per litre)

	Na^+	K^+	kJ
Isotonic saline (N/S)	153	—	—
Hartmann's solution	140	4	200 (approx.)
5% dextrose	—	—	840
Dextrose/saline (D/S)	30	—	670

Isotonic saline is often referred to as 'normal' saline; it is an aqueous solution of 0.9% NaCl; this concentration is isotonic with normal plasma, i.e. has the same osmolality. The molecular weight of NaCl is 58.5; thus the molar solution has $58.5\,g\,l^{-1}$. Normal saline solution has $9\,g\,l^{-1}$; the molar strength of saline is therefore $9/58.5 = 0.153$ molar or $153\,mmol\,l^{-1}$.

Hartmann is a contemporary paediatrician who designed his solution by adding lactate to Ringer's (the latter is similar to extracellular fluid), with the aim of treating mild metabolic acidosis. Peri-operatively it does not differ significantly in its effects from isotonic saline.

Examples of a 24 h fluid prescription for a normal 70 kg adult:

5% dextrose, isotonic saline, 5% dextrose:
   1 litre over 8 hours each, or
Dextrose/saline: 1 litre 8 hourly

General Comments

The average daily requirements stated above correspond to the normal physiological losses through the urine (1.5 l), faeces (100–200 ml), perspiration (300–500 ml) and respiration (500 ml).

Unphysiological losses may arise from: surgical drains, nasogastric tubes or vomiting, diarrhoea, excessive body temperature and excessive urinary output due to diuretic drugs. Losses arising from nasogastric tubes, drains and urine output can easily be measured in volume and in Na^+/K^+ content; vomit and diarrhoea are more difficult to measure with accuracy, and losses due to high body or ambient temperatures can only be roughly estimated.

The measurable losses must always be replaced as accurately as possible in volume, Na^+ and K^+ content; note that diarrhoea has a high K^+ content ($20–50\,mmol\,l^{-1}$) and vomit has a high chloride content ($80–100\,mmol\,l^{-1}$). Patients on thiazide diuretics or frusemide may lose $50–70\,mmol$ of K^+ per litre of urine.

Elevation of body temperature is reasonably compensated for by an increase in the normal water, Na^+ and K^+ intake of 15% for each degree C above the normal 37.

The Surgical Patient

Not all patients undergoing surgery need intravenous fluid therapy. Indeed, intravenous fluid administration is not devoid of risks (air embolism, deep vein thrombosis, overloading), discomfort to the patient, or considerable cost, so it should not be undertaken lightly.

Most intra-abdominal or intrathoracic operations, and those in the area of the mouth require at least 24 to 48 hours of total intravenous fluid replacement. Blood loss in excess of 10% of total blood volume, post-operative ileus or persistent nausea are additional indications.

If it is anticipated that the need for total intravenous replacement will last for more than 72 hours, or if the patient has dehydration, K depletion or a poor nutritional state pre-operatively, then a special regime should be instituted from the start.

During major surgery additional losses may occur due to movement of fluid from the vascular compartment into the interstitial space. This results from the trauma of surgery and leads to a deficit of functional extracellular fluid. The amount is difficult to estimate. A rough guide for fluid replacement intra-operatively (including evaporative losses) is $5–10$ ml $kg^{-1}\,h^{-1}$ of Hartmann's or isotonic saline.

Three Special Problems

(a) Dehydration

This is a common situation meaning depletion of water, nearly always accompanied by Na depletion. Clinically, the symptoms and signs are: thirst, dry mucosae, loss of elasticity of the skin, fall in urine output, collapsed veins, cold extremities and tachycardia. The important laboratory findings are a high Hb ($>16 \, g \, dl^{-1}$), high osmolality of the urine and a low central venous pressure (CVP, Chapter 14).

Isotonic saline or Hartmann's should be used for replacement at an initial rate of 1 litre in 2–4 hours, monitoring the signs listed above at hourly intervals.

(b) Potassium depletion

Chronic depletion is commonly seen in the ageing hospital population treated with diuretics for hypertension or cardiac failure. Plasma K^+ starts to fall below the normal minimum of $3.5 \, mmol \, l^{-1}$ only after 10% of total body K^+ has been lost (400 mmol). A good additional indicator of depletion is a high plasma bicarbonate value ($>28 \, mmol \, l^{-1}$) associated with an acid urine.

Depletion of 400–600 mmol causes intracellular acidosis as hydrogen ions enter the cells to maintain ionic equilibrium. Losses should be replaced over several days with oral supplements, and the underlying cause corrected.

Sometimes the patient is unable to take oral supplements, so K^+ must be given intravenously. It is administered as KCl, and concentrations of more than $20 \, mmol \, l^{-1}$ in saline or dextrose cause pain and thrombosis in peripheral veins. Rapid replacement is rarely advisable. If absolutely necessary, it may be carried out through a CVP line in the intensive care unit, with continuous ECG monitoring and frequent plasma K^+ measurements.

(c) Water intoxication

This rarely occurs, but has dramatic consequences due to hyponatraemia; the cause is usually iatrogenic. Other causes include compulsive water drinking, transurethral resection of the prostate with water irrigation and a few rare medical disorders.

Overprescription of intravenous dextrose solutions is the main cause, and this was not infrequent in labour wards. When plasma Na^+ falls rapidly to below $120 \, mmol \, l^{-1}$ mental disturbances occur, usually followed by convulsions.

Mannitol ($1 \, g \, kg^{-1}$) and frusemide ($0.5 \, mg \, kg^{-1}$) followed by 0.9% or 1.8% saline intravenously is an effective treatment of this emergency; a urinary catheter is needed.

Blood Transfusion, Bleeding Disorders and Colloid Administration

Effects of Blood Loss

If the haemoglobin (Hb) value was previously normal, blood replacement is only necessary when more than 15% of the estimated blood volume (EBV) has been lost. Until then clear fluids are substituted.

Formula for EBV:

Babies	$80 \, ml \, kg^{-1}$
Adult male	$75 \, ml \, kg^{-1}$
Female	$70 \, ml \, kg^{-1}$

In the absence of transfusion, a litre blood loss in a 70 kg adult is compensated for in 36 hours by transfer of interstitial fluid to the plasma circulating volume, red blood cells being restored in 3–5 days. Rapid loss, inadequately replaced, leads to hypovolaemia and, if excessive, to reduced cardiac output and peripheral perfusion, with hypotension and eventual organ failure.

Estimation of Blood Loss in the Surgical Patient

History and Clinical Examination

If there is acute blood loss pre-operatively, the

symptoms and signs are those of acute hypo-volaemia: thirst, dry mucosae, pallor, cold extremities, tachycardia and hypotension (Chapter 13). If the blood loss has taken place slowly over days or weeks, the symptoms and signs are those of anaemia: tiredness, dyspnoea of effort, pallor, tachycardia and tachypnoea.

Hb Level

Acute loss: in the early stages of blood loss this is unreliable, but once the patient is stable, it may be a good indication of blood requirements, i.e. $1 \, g \, dl^{-1}$ of Hb deficit is equivalent to 1 unit of blood loss in a 70 kg man.

Chronic loss: in chronic anaemia, assessment of cause (e.g. iron deficiency) is the primary step in therapy. A Hb level of $10 \, g \, dl^{-1}$ is the minimum requirement for routine surgery (4–$6 \, g \, dl^{-1}$ in haemodialysed renal patients).

Swabs

Weighing: Weight of blood-stained swab minus the dry weight of the swab equals the blood loss in grams ($1.25 \, ml$ blood g^{-1}). One unit of whole blood contains about 400 ml of blood (100 ml anti-coagulant), so if blood loss is 800 ml, this must be replaced by 2 units of blood.

Washing machine: all the swabs are placed in a washing machine (literally). The freed Hb alters the electrical conductivity of the medium thus allowing blood loss to be quantified.

Cross Matching

(a) Major blood groups

ABO grouping refers to the presence of antigen on the surface of the red blood cell (RBC). Thus 'A' blood contains 'A' antigen, 'B' blood the 'B' antigen and so on. 'O' blood contains no major RBC antigen and contains both anti-A and anti-B antibody in the serum (Table 6.2).

In an emergency, where cross matched blood is not available, O blood can be considered as 'universal donor blood'. However, it should be given as packed RBCs, so that the amount of anti-A and -B

TABLE 6.2 Distribution of major blood groups

Blood type	Antibodies present in serum	% Population in UK
O blood	anti-A and anti-B	45
A blood	anti-B	43
B blood	anti-A	7
AB blood	no anti-A or -B	5

transfused is kept to a minimum, thus limiting destruction of recipient RBCs. Similarly, people with group AB may receive other groups ('universal recipient') but again only if the transfusion is packed.

(b) Rhesus groups

Eighty five per cent of the population contain the rhesus (Rh) antigen (usually D) and are Rh positive, 15% are Rh negative. Normally, no anti-D antibody is present in blood of either group, but Rh negative patients produce anti-D antibody in response to transfusion with Rh positive blood. Thus, Rh negative blood must be given to Rh negative patients to avoid transfusion reactions in the future as well as haemolytic disease of the new born if the patient is female. Rh positive patients do not produce anti-D antibody and thus can receive either Rh negative or positive blood safely.

(c) Cross-match procedure

A suspension of donor RBCs is incubated with recipient serum at 37°C. Look for agglutination (clumping).

(d) Anticoagulants for blood storage

Acid citrate dextrose (ACD) is now little used and has been replaced by citrate phosphate dextrose with adenine (CPD A). The citrate is present in excess, and chelates calcium thus inhibiting the coagulation cascade (see page 129). If blood is given rapidly it may acutely lower ionised calcium and accentuate myocardial depression.

Storage Changes to Blood and Components

Blood is stored at 4°C. Red blood cell viability and clotting factors (except factors V and VIII) are well maintained to 35 days in CPD A. Factor V is down to 50% at two weeks, factor VIII is down to 50% in 24 hours. Platelets are reduced to 20% in 24 hours, and are major contributors to the formation of microaggregates in stored blood. To retain viability for subsequent transfusion in thrombocytopaenia, platelets must be separated immediately following collection of blood. They may then be stored at 22°C for up to 5 days, in packs equivalent to the amount contained in 8 units of fresh blood. Fresh frozen plasma (FFP) is stored at -22°C and will keep indefinitely at this temperature. It must be thawed immediately prior to use in a water bath at 37°C.

Indications for Blood Transfusion

(a) Whole blood versus packed cells

The administration of 'whole blood' as opposed to packed cells (PRBCs) is rarely indicated. It not only accumulates excess K^+, NH_4^+, acid and so on during storage, which may be dangerous in renal or hepatic disease, but the excess volume may precipitate cardiac failure in susceptible patients who are being transfused to correct chronic anaemia. In addition, if plasma is separated into its components immediately after donation, fresh frozen plasma, cryoprecipitate and platelets can be used to treat other patients who have need of such factors.

(b) When to transfuse blood

An adequate Hb concentration must be maintained to ensure adequate tissue oxygen delivery (Chapter 12). This can only be achieved by increasing cardiac output if the Hb is less than $10\,\mathrm{g\,dl^{-1}}$ (the minimum level which should exist in the surgical or critically ill patient). During surgery, a blood loss equal to 10% EBV (e.g.

450 ml) is replaced with Hartmann's or 0.9% saline, as blood loss of this amount is well tolerated. As much of this fluid leaves the circulation to replace transferred interstitial fluid, it is often given in larger volumes than the amount of blood lost. Once blood loss exceeds 15% of EBV, it must be replaced by PRBCs, as Hb then approaches the minimum level of $10\,\mathrm{g\,dl^{-1}}$. Replacement of blood loss between 10 and 20% of EBV is a matter of clinical discretion.

In the traumatised patient where measurement of blood loss is difficult or impossible, replacement is determined clinically and by frequent haematocrit determinations.

(c) How to transfuse blood

An adequate sized cannula (and vein) is mandatory if rapid blood transfusion is anticipated (see page 21). Blood is stored at 4°C so it should be warmed to 37°C prior to infusion, especially if this is rapid, to avoid the risk of cold-induced cardiac dysrhythmias and overall cooling of the patient. Specially designed, purpose built, thermostatically controlled warmers must be used; under no circumstances should blood be warmed in 'hot water' as inadequate temperature control may cause protein degeneration. In addition, storage of blood in CPD A is now extended to 5 weeks, so the amount of microaggregates (of platelets, white cells and red cells) is markedly increased. The incidence of pulmonary microvascular lesions may be reduced by the use of 20 to 40 μm filters which are placed between the bag and giving set.

The viscosity of blood (particularly if PRBCs and cold) makes rapid transfusion difficult. This is overcome by inserting the blood pack inside a special bag pressurised up to 300 mmHg.

Use of Plasma Component Therapy

Transfusion of stored blood (whole or PRBCs) in excess of about 50% of EBV leads to dilution of clotting factors V and VIII and inhibitors such as anti-thrombin III (AT III). The latter is important for coagulation control; depletion during major surgery and blood loss leads to an increased risk of thrombosis. Administration of FFP obviates these problems by supplying factors V and VIII together with AT III. It should be given at a rate of 2 units per 10 units of blood transfused. It is unusual for the platelet count to be reduced to critical levels ($<50\,000$ mm^{-3}) until the EBV has been replaced (approximately 10 units in the average adult).

Diagnosis and Treatment of Bleeding (Surgery and ICU)

It is obviously essential to exclude surgical causes of bleeding before exhaustive coagulation studies are undertaken.

Tests for the diagnosis of bleeding in the surgical patient

1 Whole blood coagulation time (WBCT) can be performed at the bedside or in theatre. A sample of blood (5 ml) is placed in a plain glass bottle, kept at body temperature and observed for the presence of clot. This should occur in 5 to 15 minutes followed by retraction in 30 to 60 minutes. If this test is normal, bleeding is unlikely to be due to an acquired coagulopathy. Clot which initially forms and then dissolves is usually due to excessive fibrinolysis either primary or secondary. A weak, friable clot is seen in hypofibrinogenaemia.

2 Prothrombin time (PT, one stage 12–14 seconds or ratio with control 0.9–1.2) is an indicator of the levels of factors I, II, V, VII and X. It depends on the addition of thromboplastin and therefore assesses the extrinsic pathway of coagulation, particularly factor VII. It is prolonged in liver disease, vitamin K deficiency, massive blood transfusion, warfarin anticoagulation, high-dose heparin therapy and disseminated intravascular coagulation (DIC).

3 Activated partial thromboplastin time (aPTT, normally 24–28 s) is an indicator of the levels of factor V and VIII. It depends on the addition of phospholipid and therefore assesses the intrinsic pathway of coagulation. It is prolonged following massive transfusion, haemophilia, heparin and high-dose warfarin anticoagulation and DIC.

4 Activated coagulation time (ACT). A simple automated machine is available to perform this test which relies on surface activation of clotting by diatomaceous earth. It thus depends to a certain extent on normal platelet triggered coagulation as well as the factors mentioned above. The normal value is 80–110 seconds, and is prolonged in heparin therapy, for which it is used as a monitor in renal units and in cardiac surgery.

5 Platelet count (normally $>200\,000$ mm^{-3}) is reduced by dilutional massive transfusion and in DIC. Spontaneous bleeding may occur at levels below $100\,000$ mm^{-3} and always if below $50\,000$ mm^{-3}. Platelet function may be affected by aspirin and similar drugs, but the count remains normal. Penicillin may be toxic to platelets, especially if used in high doses in the critically ill.

6 Fibrinogen titre (normally 200–400 mg dl^{-1}) reduction in the critically ill patient is usually dilutional or as a result of fibrinolysis. The latter may be primary due to plasminogen activation (sepsis) but is usually secondary to DIC.

7 Bleeding time (normally less than 7 minutes) prolongation with normal coagulation studies and platelet count is usually due to platelet dysfunction.

8 Thrombin time (normally 15–30 s) measures the conversion of fibrinogen into fibrin, by addition of thrombin to the blood sample. It is prolonged with gross deviations of the fibrinogen/fibrin degradation products (FDPs) and heparin. In the absence of heparin it is a sensitive monitor of the presence of FDPs.

9 Fibrin degradation products (FDPs, normally <16 μg ml^{-1}) are formed by the action of plasmin on fibrin clot. They are formed in excess following major trauma, haemorrhage and tissue destruction, or from excessive fibrinolytic activity. FDPs in excessive quantities produce anticoagulation by inhibition of fibrin formation and platelet aggregation, and also increase vascular permeability.

Differential diagnosis

Differential diagnosis of the most frequent causes of bleeding are outlined Table 6.3. Apart from the dilutional effects of massive transfusion, other common causes are:

1 Disseminated intravascular coagulation (DIC) may occur from: trauma, burns, haemolytic transfusion reaction, sepsis, profound hypotension and amniotic fluid embolus. Treatment is directed to the cause, but symptomatic replacement of clotting factors is essential. Reduction in excessive coagulation is sometimes treated with heparin.
2 Isolated thrombocytopaenia appearing in the critically ill patient is usually due to a drug effect, such as penicillin. Aspirin and dipyridamole do not cause thrombocytopaenia, so the diagnosis is confirmed by platelet function tests which will be abnormal. It must be treated by withdrawal of the drug and administration of platelet concentrates.
3 Liver disease results in coagulopathy for the reason that the liver is the sole source of all the clotting factors (except possibly factor VIII).

Factors II (prothrombin), VII, IX and X are vitamin K dependent which is poorly absorbed in obstructive jaundice due to the absence of bile salts in the intestine. Platelet count is often low due to hypersplenism.

4 Excess warfarin in unstable anticoagulation control leads initially to an increase in PT followed by a raised aPTT. In patients in whom surgery is contemplated, the PT ratio should not exceed 2:1. This should be corrected with FFP or very small doses of vitamin K (1 mg), larger doses will reverse anticoagulation for many days and thus predispose the patient to thrombosis.
5 Excess heparin in unstable anticoagulation control leads initially to an increase in aPTT, ACT and thrombin time. Subsequently, PT is also prolonged. It is easily reversed by administration of protamine sulphate i.v. with close monitoring of ACT

Colloid Administration

Following major haemorrhage, but prior to availability of cross-matched blood, circulating

TABLE 6.3 Test results in bleeding diatheses: possible cause of bleeding

Test	Massive transfusion	DIC	Primary fibrinolysis	Platelet dysfunction	Liver disease	Excess warfarin/heparin
WBCT	∧	∧∧	∧∧	N	∧	∧∧/∧∧
PT	∧	∧∧	∧∧	N	∧∧∧	∧∧∧/∧
aPTT	∧	∧∧	∧∧	N	∧	∧/∧∧∧
ACT	∧	∧	∧	∧	∧	∧/∧∧∧
Platelets	∨	∨∨∨	N	N/∨∨∨	N/∨	N
Fibrinogen	∨	∨∨∨	∨	N	∨	N
Bleeding Time	∧∧	∧∧∧	∧∧∧	∧∧	∧/∧∧	∧∧∧
Thrombin Time	∧	∧∧∧	∧∧∧	N	∧	N or ∧
FDPs (μg ml^{-1})	<16	>32	>16	N	<16	N

Key ∧ = raised or prolonged   ∨ = low   N = normal
∧∧ = markedly raised or prolonged   ∨∨ = very low
∧∧∧ = extremely raised or prolonged   ∨∨∨ = extremely low

volume must be maintained. This is achieved by infusion of 'clear fluids' such as Hartmann's solution or 0.9% saline. However, if blood loss is severe, excessive volumes of these fluids (more than 2 litres) may be required to maintain a minimum cardiac output. This is because they are isotonic 'crystalloid' solutions which exert no colloid oncotic pressure (COP) and thus are freely distributed throughout the extracellular fluid volume (ECF). This may lead to a reduction in COP in blood with interstitial and pulmonary oedema.

Fluids which are isotonic, but also exert COP (due to the presence of molecules of size 30 000–60 000 Daltons) are called 'colloids'. They may be derived from blood products, such as plasma protein fraction (PPF) or human albumin (5% or 20%), or they may be derived from non-human material, such as dextrans (40 or 70), gelatin (Gelofusin R and Haemaccel R) and hydroxyethyl starch (Hetastarch R). They have a much longer half-life in the circulation compared to crystalloids (3 to 24 hours) as opposed to 15 minutes), so less volume is required to maintain circulating volume, and there is less risk of oedema. However, they have disadvantages in that they are expensive, particularly human blood products, or may cause allergic reactions. Dextrans may also interfere with blood coagulation and cross matching, and in certain circumstances Dextran 40 may block the renal tubules and precipitate acute renal failure.

In general, crystalloids should be used first for resuscitation, unless it is believed that the arrival of cross-matched blood will be delayed.

Hazards and Complications of Blood Transfusion

Although in the UK blood transfusion is a relatively safe procedure it should never be undertaken lightly and only when really indicated (as above). Major transfusion reactions characterised by a severe anaphylactic response (Chapter 13) result from ABO incompatibility, e.g. a group B patient with anti-A antibodies receiving A positive donor blood. This usually results from administrative errors and is rare. The effects are often very serious, leading to severe hypotension and organ failure. The transfusion must be stopped as soon as possible and appropriate measures taken. Less serious minor 'allergic' reactions occur more frequently due to the presence of non-red cell antibody/antigen reactions. Itching, fever, urticaria and occasionally bronchospasm and hypotension characterise these reactions which may be treated with anti-histamines and by stopping the transfusion if necessary. Viral (e.g. hepatitis B and AIDS) and microbial transmission is very unusual, thanks to effective screening of donors and blood. Fluid overload is still one of the commonest hazards of blood transfusion.

7

Accidents and complications of anaesthesia

Fatal Accidents

A high proportion of fatal accidents are related to inadvertent misconnections of pipes and tubes, or wrong gas flows in the anaesthetic machine. Some 16% are related to inexperience of the anaesthetist. At the top of the list of causes of death are: iatrogenic cardiovascular depression or hypovolaemia, post-operative respiratory depression secondary to neuromuscular blockade and opiates, difficult intubations, and inadequate post-operative care. Fatalities following the unskilled administration of local anaesthetics, mostly Bier's blocks given in accident and emergency departments by non-anaesthetists, are on the increase.

Common Complications: Causes and Treatment

Complications may arise at induction of anaesthesia, during maintenance and in the post-operative period. Only the commonest will be discussed.

(a) Complications at induction

1 Changes in blood pressure happen in nearly all inductions; a 10–20 mmHg drop in systolic blood pressure is taken as a 'normal response', and a more severe drop is usually due to overdose (relative or absolute) of anaesthetic or hypovolaemia. Treatment includes rapid administration of intravenous fluid and head-down position. Occasionally a vasopressor drug (e.g. ephedrine) is needed.

Anaphylaxis (Chapter 13) is a much rarer cause of hypotension following induction of anaesthesia; it is treated with i.v. fluids together with adrenaline 1 mg subcutaneously (or 10 μg i.v. boluses if ECG monitor available) which also relieves bronchospasm, if present.

Hypertension is common following laryngoscopy and intubation, but leads to complications only if there is ischaemic heart disease or raised intracranial pressure; beta-blockers or i.v. lignocaine are effective in prevention.

2 Vomiting or regurgitation of stomach contents is a feared complication in emergency and obstetric surgery; a 'rapid sequence induction' is indicated (Chapter 8).

3 In spontaneous ventilation anaesthesia without intubation, cough and laryngeal spasm are troublesome and occur mainly in unpremedicated patients before adequate surgical anaesthesia is reached.

4 Intubation may be difficult or impossible, or may be complicated with broken teeth or vocal cord injury.

5 The intravenous agent may accidentally be injected subcutaneously or intra-arterially. Thiopentone (2.5%) subcutaneously is not serious, but intra-arterial injection leads to severe pain and possible loss of a hand or finger. Treatment includes local application of hyaluronidase to increase absorption if subcutaneous, and intra-arterial injection of procaine if the needle is still in situ.

6 If regional anaesthesia is used, systemic side effects of the local anaesthetic drug are common, such as loss of consciousness, respiratory and cardiac depression, and convulsions.

Epidural and subarachnoid (spinal) anaesthesia is nearly always complicated by a drop of blood pressure that can be attenuated with prior administration of i.v. fluids; if this is ineffective, ephedrine in 5 mg i.v. boluses may be added.

Dural or blood taps are additional complications of epidurals. Dural taps often cause severe headaches starting within 24 hours of the tap and lasting for days or even weeks, due to leakage of cerebrospinal fluid through the hole made in the dura by the needle. They occur on sitting or standing and usually are totally incapacitating. The treatment consists of non-steroidal analgesics, administration of additional fluids and rest in the horizontal position; if persistent they can be effectively treated with an injection of 10–20 ml of autologous blood ('blood patch') into the epidural space.

More rarely the level of sensory and motor block is too high ('total spinal') causing respiratory muscle paralysis requiring mechanical ventilation.

(b) Complications during maintenance of anaesthesia

1 Dysrhythmias occur frequently; they include tachycardia, bradycardia and ectopic beats; they are usually due to inadequate analgesia, carbon dioxide retention or hypovolaemia (Chapter 4).
2 Hypotension is usually the result of either hypovolaemia or overdose of anaesthetic or other drugs with hypotensive effects (e.g. droperidol, tubocurarine, morphine). Hypertension usually results from too light anaesthesia, but occasionally is present in spite of adequate anaesthesia. It may respond to propranolol and a small dose of an hypotensive drug (e.g. hydrallazine or trimetaphan).
3 Disconnections or misconnections of tubes and ventilators are common. The properly trained anaesthetist checks and knows his apparatus; like the airline pilot, he should run regular (say 30 s intervals) eye checks on the patient and equipment during the anaesthetic.
4 More rare complications during maintenance are hypothermia (Chapter 15), pulmonary embolism with air or thrombi, patient awareness, transfusion reactions (Chapter 6), pneumothorax, and malignant hyperthermia.

(c) Post-operative complications

(1) *Recovery or immediate complications* (first few minutes after discontinuing the anaesthetic):

Shivering does not require specific treatment, oxygen should be given because of increased consumption.

If vomiting occurs the patient should be turned on the side, head down and airway cleared. Unless contraindicated, all patients should be turned on their side after operation.

Laryngeal spasm on removing endotracheal tube usually resolves with 100% oxygen under slight pressure.

Failure to wake up or failure to breathe is either too deep anaesthesia, excessive narcotic analgesia, muscle paralysis, or hypocarbia; it may rarely be the result of hypoglycaemia or a cerebral ischaemic accident during surgery.

(2) *Possible late complications are many:*

Nausea and vomiting are the most common and are dealt with in Chapter 5.

Respiratory depression is also common and that is why oxygen therapy is indicated post-operatively (Chapter 12). The effects of the anaesthetic agents, analgesics and muscle relaxants all contribute. Patients should leave the recovery area only after being assessed by the anaesthetist.

Pulmonary complications are relatively common, due to accumulation of secretions. This results from the presence of pain and to depression of the cough reflex by analgesics. Susceptible patients (Chapter 2) should have physiotherapy instituted post-operatively.

Urinary retention is more common following epidural or spinal anaesthesia and may require short-term catheterisation. Morphine may precipitate acute retention in men with adenoma of the prostate.

Muscular pains are frequent as a result of suxamethonium administration, more so in young muscular men. A non-opiate analgesic may provide relief.

Serious neurological complications are fortunately rare, but varied.

Transient headache following a general anaesthetic is common and usually self-limiting. Following dural tap, headaches are frequent and difficult to treat (see above).

Convulsions are very rare in non-epileptics, and the most likely causes are water intoxication or extreme hypoxia.

Peripheral nerve injuries may occur as a result of inappropriate positioning of the patient during surgery, e.g. brachial plexus lesions, facial nerve and lateral popliteal nerve palsies (Chapter 4).

Following epidural anaesthesia a localised persistence of sensory block or muscle weakness may be found, and usually resolves spontaneously within 30 days.

Coarse voice or vocal cord palsy may complicate uneventful intubation and may be prolonged. The cause is unknown.

The cornea of the eye may be damaged because the eyelids were not taped shut during surgery.

Finally, joints are easy to dislocate, particularly in paralysed patients. The hip may be dislocated on moving to or from lithotomy position, and the shoulder may be dislocated on turning the unconscious patient. The jaw bone is often reversibly dislocated on trying to maintain an airway.

8
Specialised anaesthesia

Certain types of surgery demand special skills from the anaesthetist, in order to provide ideal operating conditions. It is fair to say that all types of specialised surgery have their peculiarities as to the ideal choice of anaesthetic technique. Some demand special training such as anaesthesia for obstetric surgery, paediatric surgery, neurosurgery and cardiothoracic surgery. Hypotensive anaesthesia is applied in special circumstances. Day case and casualty department surgery are also discussed as they are of special interest for the readers of this book.

Obstetric Anaesthesia

There are special considerations with respect to the welfare of the fetus or new-born baby, and to the safety of the mother.

(a) The fetus

If a pregnant woman must have an operation, effects of drugs and cardiovascular or respiratory disturbances associated with anaesthesia should be taken into account.

The state of fetal development is important; in the first six weeks of pregnancy the effects of drugs upon the formation of organs and limbs must be considered. The well-tested drugs have proven safe in this respect, such as nitrous oxide, halothane, thiopentone and pethidine. Neuromuscular blockers do not cross the placental barrier easily, so pancuronium or suxamethonium may be used. Newly introduced drugs should be avoided.

The anaesthetic technique must be such that the oxygen delivery and perfusion of the preg-nant uterus is not compromised at any stage. For example, the pregnant patient under anaesthesia should not be kept supine without a wedge under the right buttock or a tilt of the table to avoid vena caval (or aortic) compression by the weight of the pregnant uterus.

(b) The new-born baby

If anaesthesia is administered just before delivery, as for caesarean section, then the effects of the drugs upon the new-born baby must be considered. With the exception of neuromuscular blockers, all other anaesthetic agents readily cross into the placental circulation.

Induction agents such as thiopentone have only mild effects if given in the usual dosage of 4–5 mg kg^{-1} of maternal body weight. The premature or retarded growth baby is considerably more affected. Narcotic analgesics frequently have a marked effect on the new-born, particularly after normal vaginal delivery without general anaesthesia, when pethidine or another narcotic is given for pain relief within two hours of delivery. They have depressant effects upon the new-born, particularly upon respiratory drive, which can be reliably reversed with naloxone.

All other depressant drugs, including sedatives, antiemetics, beta-blockers and local anaesthetics, have a potential danger with regard to the new-born, especially if premature.

(c) The mother

The pregnant woman at term is at special risk from induction of general anaesthesia because of an increased risk of passive regurgitation of acid stomach contents (pH is often <2, and volume increased in pregnancy). Inhalation of quantities as small as 10 ml may cause a fatal aspiration pneumonia known as the Mendelson syndrome. The administration of antacids and histamine 2 blockers pre-operatively, and a 'rapid sequence induction' technique (see Emergency Surgery) have been recommended for some years; unfortunately, these measures have not had a beneficial effect upon the national figures for mortality. The experience of the anaesthetist and of his assistant seems to be the most important factor in determining mortality.

Epidural anaesthesia does not have a safer record for the mother in the national figures. In experienced hands it is a preferable method for both mother and new-born, provided that both surgeon and patient are cooperative.

There are special considerations with regard to obstetric complications such as pre-eclampsia and amniotic fluid embolism, that are outside the scope of this book.

(d) Obstetric analgesia

There are several methods available to alleviate labour pains. Most obstetric units adopt a flexible policy as to the method to be used first, usually allowing the expectant mother to choose. The majority are given intramuscular pethidine (75–100 mg two hourly), usually supplemented by Entonox (50% N_2O in O_2); the latter must be self administered via a special demand valve necessitating a snug fit of the mask round the face to operate efficiently. This prevents overdosage as the patient lets go of the mask when drowsy. Application should be confined to the duration of each contraction. The combined pethidine–Entonox method is effective in 20–30% of women. Lumbar epidural analgesia is more effective (60–80%). Having established an intravenous infusion of isotonic saline or Hartmann's solution, an 18G catheter is introduced into the epidural space, usually at L3–4, as described in Chapter 18. After a test dose of 2–3 ml, 8–10 ml of 0.25% plain bupivacaine is injected via the catheter. The blood pressure must be monitored at 5 minute intervals for 20 minutes, and the level of the block ascertained at 15 minute intervals for the first hour. The

object of the test dose is to ensure that the small amount injected does not cause immediate (within 3 minutes) blocking effects suggesting subarachnoid placement of the catheter (See page 52). A fall of systolic blood pressure to 90 mmHg (or lower) must be rapidly treated to avoid compromising uterine perfusion. Treatment consists of:

1 intravenous fluid administration
2 positioning the patient in the lateral position with head down tilt
3 if necessary, 5 mg boluses of ephedrine injected intravenously, at three minute intervals, up to a maximum of 30 mg.

Specially trained midwives may top-up the epidural at hourly intervals, and the concentration of bupivacaine may be increased to 0.375% (equal volumes of 0.25 and 0.5% mixed) if the first dose of 0.25% proved too short acting or only partially effective.

Paediatric Anaesthesia

This encompasses all ages from new-born to 16 years. Only the problems relating to the small child and new-born will be outlined.

(a) Neonatal surgery

Surgery performed in the first 28 days of life poses special problems on several fronts.

First, the size of the patient renders most of the ordinary equipment useless. Special laryngoscopes and lightweight tubes and connectors must be available. Venous cannulation is especially difficult, and the usual manoeuvres of intubation and monitoring of the patient need special training.

Secondly, the response of the new-born to some anaesthetic agents is different: it is enhanced and prolonged with narcotic analgesics and local anaesthetics, or reduced with some neuromuscular blockers.

Thirdly, the homeostatic systems of the new-born function at a different level. There is a much larger body surface area to weight ratio which leads to a proportionately higher cardiac output, oxygen consumption and fluid requirement; temperature control is also much more precarious. It must be a constant preoccupation of the anaesthetist to maintain body temperature during anaesthesia. Maintenance of the fluid balance also requires special training for assessment and for therapy.

Most operations performed in neonates are for correction of congenital defects that need urgent intervention such as severe cardiac malformations, diaphragmatic hernia, omphalocele, tracheo-oesophageal fistula and pyloric stenosis.

(b) Surgery in the small child

The same comments as for the neonate apply with regard to the differences in homeostasis as compared with the adult, but to a lesser degree. The response and elimination of anaesthetic drugs is comparable to the adult.

Additional problems of the small child relate to the psychological aspects of surgery and induction of anaesthesia. The most important factor in determining a smooth induction is perhaps a calm unhurried atmosphere in the anaesthetic room.

Neurosurgical Anaesthesia

The special requirements of anaesthesia for neurosurgery are mainly concerned with the effects of anaesthetic technique upon intracranial pressure, the major determinants of which are the arterial blood pressure, arterial carbon dioxide tension, temperature and the anaesthetic agents used. Narcotic analgesics are best avoided for premedication, due to their respiratory depressant effect with consequent rise in $PaCO_2$.

At induction of anaesthesia, intubation usually causes a substantial rise in arterial pressure thereby also increasing intracranial pressure. This can be effectively prevented by previous administration of propranolol or lignocaine intravenously, and an adequate dose of thiopentone ($6 \, mg \, kg^{-1}$).

During operation, the blood pressure must be kept at a normal or hypotensive level. A reduction of systolic blood pressure to 60 mmHg

may be required for short periods (e.g. for clipping an aneurysm); this is best achieved with a sodium nitroprusside infusion. Direct monitoring of arterial blood pressure through an intra-arterial cannula is desirable.

If the patient is in the sitting position for posterior fossa surgery there is considerable risk of air embolism; special monitoring must be available as this complication may be fatal. Monitoring of end-tidal carbon dioxide (this falls transiently but obviously if more than 20 ml of air is trapped in the pulmonary circulation) or the use of a precordial stethoscope or ultrasound detector (air bubbles passing through the right ventricle can be heard) is mandatory. Respiratory depression post-operatively must be avoided; the use of narcotic analgesics during and after the operation should be kept to a minimum (in some centres they are not used at all), and adequate recovery from the neuromuscular block must be ensured.

Cardiothoracic Anaesthesia
(a) Cardiac anaesthesia

There has been an increase in vein graft surgery for coronary artery disease in recent years. The frequency of operations to correct acquired valve defects has declined, and that for congenital defects has remained approximately constant.

The main anaesthetic problems are related to poor cardiac reserve. Anaesthetic techniques must be such that the use of drugs with a depressant effect upon the heart is kept to a minimum. If the cardiac output is fixed, as in aortic stenosis, the peripheral resistance must not be severely decreased. Drugs with a marked effect upon peripheral resistance such as morphine and tubocurarine must be used with great caution; fentanyl and pancuronium, that do not release histamine, are preferable.

Special monitoring is needed for surgery such as continuous arterial pressure, blood-gases, right atrial pressure, core temperature and urine output. The first three are usually done through percutaneously inserted cannuli in the radial artery and right internal jugular (or subclavian) vein.

The aspects of whole body cooling and maintenance of extra-corporeal circulation are outside the scope of this book.

(b) Thoracic anaesthesia

Anaesthesia for surgery of the lung and oesophagus also requires special techniques. Normally one lung or part of a lung will be collapsed during surgery and a special double-lumen endotracheal tube may be needed to ventilate each lung separately. There is a choice of various models of these tubes, which can be right sided or left sided depending upon which lung is to be collapsed during surgery.

One lung ventilation has its problems: it is advisable to use higher than usual inspired concentrations of oxygen (some even use 100%) to maintain PaO_2 above 10 kPa (75 mmHg).

Other difficulties may arise with large amounts of secretions or pus, or with the presence of bronchopleural fistulae, which merit individually tailored anaesthetic techniques.

Hypotensive Anaesthesia

It was mentioned under neurosurgery that blood pressure reduction may be beneficial during part of the operation. Other types of surgery may also be facilitated by hypotension. Examples are plastic and middle ear surgery, but in these instances the blood pressure should be kept down for most of the procedure rather than just for a short period.

Hypotension provides the surgeon with a bloodless field in which he can operate much more rapidly, with benefit to the patient. Arterial blood pressure is not the only factor: positioning the patient correctly, adequate analgesia and avoidance of hypercarbia are just as important.

The anaesthetic technique includes drugs that tend to lower the blood pressure such as tubocurarine as a muscle relaxant and morphine as an analgesic. Administration of a beta-blocker before any specific hypotensive agent is used greatly reduces the requirements by abolishing reflex tachycardia. The specific hypotensive agents are therefore kept only for fine moment to moment adjustment of the pressure. Sodium nitroprusside may be used but is probably best kept for short procedures where a brief reduction in pressure is needed. Ganglion blocking agents such as pentolinium (Ansolysen, long acting) or trimetaphan (Arfonad, short acting) are preferable.

The definition of hypotension in this context is only relative to the patient's own normal blood pressure. Usually the aim is to lower the systolic pressure to approximately 50% of the pre-operative value (or 60–70 mmHg, whichever is the greater). Patients with cardiopulmonary, cerebral or renal disease must be excluded.

The techniques of blood pressure control just described may be successfully applied outside the context of anaesthesia, such as the management of severe pre-eclampsia or hypertensive emergencies.

Anaesthesia for Day Case and Emergency Surgery

Casualty officers, house surgeons and general practitioners normally deal with the pre-anaesthetic preparations or with the anaesthetic complications associated with this type of surgery.

Day case surgery

This is on the increase because funds for hospital beds are in short supply. Most deal with procedures such as cystoscopies, minor gynaecology, dental extractions and minor general surgical procedures.

Patients must be carefully selected, excluding any form of medical condition which may complicate the anaesthetic or the recovery (Chapter 2). A responsible person must help the patient return home and keep observation for at least the following 12 hours, with clear instructions about what to do if complications arise. Day patients are rarely heavily premedicated, but small children benefit from a sedative given at home on the morning of surgery in the form of a syrup, thus avoiding some of the apprehension.

There is nothing noteworthy about the anaesthetic technique except that intubation of the trachea and the use of long-acting drugs (e.g. morphine, pancuronium) is inadvisable.

Post-operatively, headaches and nausea are common and are best treated only with bed rest since they are self limiting.

If the trachea was intubated, laryngeal oedema and airway obstruction is possible, particularly in children, so the responsible accompanying person must be duly instructed in this respect.

Emergency surgery

Inevitably, emergency surgery is necessary in patients who have eaten or drunk recently. If the surgical condition can wait, it must be for long enough to ensure an empty stomach at the onset of anaesthesia. At least 6 hours should elapse since the last food or drink, and it should be remembered that the injured patient in pain retains food in the stomach for much longer. Stomach emptying may be hastened by the administration of metoclopramide (Maxolon) in a single intramuscular dose of 0.15 mg kg^{-1}, provided it is given at least half an hour prior to the administration of any narcotic analgesic or atropine (which block the gastric effects of metoclopramide).

If the operation is life saving and the patient has to be anaesthetised with a full stomach the technique of 'rapid sequence induction' must be used.

Rapid sequence induction:
1 Pre-oxygenation for 3 minutes with 100% oxygen.
2 Pressure applied to the cricoid cartilage by an experienced helper, to prevent passive regurgitation of stomach contents into the oropharynx (Sellick's manoeuvre).
3 Thiopentone, suxamethonium and intubation with a cuffed tube, having a good sucker at hand.
NB Inflation of the lungs by face mask after suxamethonium but prior to intubation is inadvisable in spite of cricoid pressure (pre-oxygenation is used to maintain PaO$_2$ for this period).

Once the patient is intubated it is advisable to aspirate the stomach contents.

Finally, it should be noted that the use of local anaesthesia does not always mean that the rules regarding stomach contents should be dispensed with. Toxic side effects of local anaesthetics include convulsions, respiratory depression and a state of general anaesthesia. A regrettable number of deaths have occurred following intravenous (Bier's) blocks of the arm due to these effects, sometimes compounded with aspiration of gastric contents.

9

Blood gases; arterial puncture

Acid–base Balance

The role of hydrogen ion (H^+ or proton) in living cells is as important as that of sodium or potassium. Its intracellular concentration has not been reliably measured in most mammalian tissues (except erythrocytes), but it is thought to be critically important. It is affected by such factors as its extracellular concentration and the trans-membrane balance of potassium ions.

Hydrogen ions are constantly produced (about $15\,mol\,day^{-1}$) by metabolism and additional amounts are ingested with food. There must be a balance between production and excretion. Some 80% ($12\,mol\,day^{-1}$) is eliminated through the lung as carbon dioxide and water, and the rest through the kidney ($3\,mol\,day^{-1}$).

The human body has several built-in mechanisms to maintain the extracellular concentration of hydrogen ion within narrow limits, namely $35–45\,nmol\,l^{-1}$ (pH 7.45–7.35). In blood, sustained concentrations above $100\,nmol\,l^{-1}$ (pH < 7.0) or below $10\,nmol\,l^{-1}$ (pH > 8.0) are incompatible with life.

(a) Regulatory mechanisms

There are two major regulatory mechanisms which tend to keep the hydrogen ion concentration at the physiological 'set point' of $40\,nmol\,l^{-1}$ (pH 7.4): a fast mechanism operated via the lung and a slow one operated via the kidney.

(1) *Respiratory homeostatic mechanisms*

The immediate determinant of hydrogen ion concentration in blood is the partial pressure of carbon dioxide (PCO_2), which is acutely dependent on pulmonary ventilation.

In a mechanically ventilated subject, the relationship between minute ventilation and the partial pressure of carbon dioxide in arterial blood ($PaCO_2$) is a curve close to a hyperbola, varying its shape with the metabolic consumption (Fig. 9.1). Note that the same increase in minute ventilation produces a much smaller fall in $PaCO_2$ at lower values.

An excess of H^+ in arterial blood stimulates both the peripheral chemoreceptors in the carotid bifurcation and the respiratory neurons in the brain stem. This causes an increase in ventilation which leads to a fall in PCO_2 and $[H^+]$ in blood, closing the negative feedback loop of this regulation. It should be noted that chemoreceptors are also stimulated by an increase in $PaCO_2$. The arterial chemoreceptors are independently stimulated by (PaO_2) values below 8 kPa (60 mmHg); the three stimuli interact with each other in a multiplicative way.

Carbon dioxide and hydrogen ion are interrelated through the reaction of the former with water to form carbonic acid; the latter dissociates into hydrogen H^+ and bicarbonate HCO_3^- ions, a major buffer system in blood.

$CO_2 + H_2O \rightleftharpoons H_2CO_3$
(catalysed by carbonic anhydrase)
$H_2CO_3 \qquad \rightleftharpoons HCO_3^- + H^+$

$K = [HCO_3^-] \times [H^+]/[H_2CO_3]$ (mass-equation)

([ ] denotes concentration and K is a proportionality factor)

Traditionally, hydrogen ion concentration has been measured in pH units, pH being the negative logarithm (base 10) of the hydrogen ion concentration $[H^+]$. Its quantitative relationship

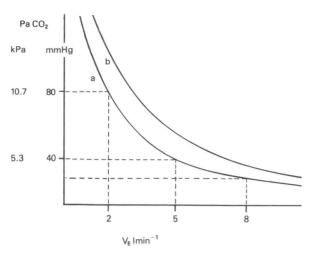

Fig. 9.1 Approximate relationship between minute ventilation (V_E) and $PaCO_2$, at two metabolic rates (b > a), in a mechanically ventilated subject

to PCO_2 is obtained by manipulation of the mass-equation shown above.

Because many phenomena relating to buffering are interpreted graphically, and the response of the H^+ electrode is logarithmic, the pH scale has proved more convenient.

$$pH = pKa + \log [HCO_3^-]/(a \times PCO_2)$$

where pKa is 6.1, and a the CO_2 solubility factor (0.03, if $PaCO_2$ is measured in mmHg, 0.2 if in kPa)

The latter is known as the Henderson–Hasselbalch equation. It has three variables, pH, $[HCO_3^-]$ and PCO_2. Thus it cannot be represented by a single curve, but rather by a family of curves forming a 'surface'.

Various authors represented this relationship in different ways: Davenport chose to plot pH against $[HCO_3^-]$ at different $PaCO_2$ values (Fig. 9.2). Sigaard–Andersen plotted pH against $PaCO_2$ at various $[HCO_3^-]$ values.

These plots were of great practical value before the era of electronic calculators to estimate the $[HCO_3^-]$ and the amount of excess acid or base present in blood. Most blood-gas machines in clinical use now have a microcomputer incorporated that instantly calculates these derived variables.

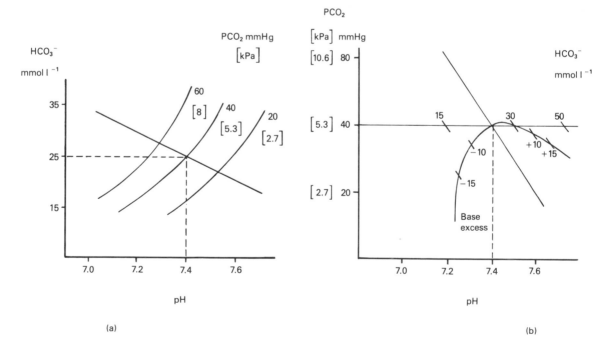

Fig. 9.2 Two ways of plotting the Henderson–Hasselbalch equation. (a) The plot of Davenport. (b) Sigaard-Andersen's plot. The straight lines in both plots are the buffer curves for whole blood with an Hb of 15 g dl^{-1}

The way each variable in the Henderson–Hasselbalch equation depends on each other is a predictable function of temperature, concentration of Hb (buffer) and Hb saturation. This is also taken into account by the computer in the blood-gas machine.

Temperature is not measured but the blood sample is warmed (or cooled) to 37°C in the measuring cuvette.

The print out of most blood-gas machines shows 8 or more results, four from direct measurement (pH, PCO_2, PO_2 and Hb), and the others derived by calculation. The latter include base excess, bicarbonate, standard bicarbonate and Hb saturation. Base excess is a calculation of the amount of acid (HCl), or base (NaOH), that would need to be added to a litre of blood (*in vitro*) to titrate the pH back to 7.40 at a PCO_2 of 5.3 kPa (40 mmHg) and at 37°C. The base excess result is negative in acidosis (it is really a 'base deficit', since NaOH would be added) and positive in alkalosis (HCl added).

The standard bicarbonate is a calculation of the bicarbonate value if the blood were to be equilibrated with a PCO_2 of 5.3 kPa (40 mmHg). It is important to be aware that only PCO_2, pH and PO_2 are obtained by direct measurement.

(2) *Renal homeostatic mechanisms*
One of the many functions of the kidney is to excrete hydrogen ions. The [H^+] in urine may be as high as 30 000 $nmol\,l^{-1}$ (pH 4.5), 800 times that of plasma. At such high [H^+], the total quantity of H^+ that can be excreted in the urine depends on its buffering power.

Two main buffer systems exist in urine: the phosphate system and the ammonia/ammonium system:

$$H_2PO_4^- \quad \rightleftharpoons H^+ + HPO_4^{2-} \ (pK = 6.8)$$
$$NH_3 + H^+ \rightleftharpoons NH_4^+ \qquad (pK = 5)$$

Note that these only work as buffers in the region of their respective pKs. The renal synthesis of ammonia is subject to regulation. Normally about 30 mmol of ammonium are excreted per day; after three days of severe acidosis as much as 200 mmol may be excreted per day. The excretion of each H^+ ion into the urine leads to reabsorption of a sodium ion, and is dependent upon the local PCO_2 and availability of carbonic anhydrase. The potassium ion competes with H^+ in urinary excretion; K^+ depletion leads to urinary loss of H^+ and alkalosis, and acidosis leads to K^+ retention and hyperkalaemia. The kidney also compensates for alkalosis by excreting excess bicarbonate; it is more effective in metabolic alkalosis because the respiratory compensation leads to an increased $PaCO_2$.

(b) Acid–base disturbances
It is important to understand the time course of acid–base disturbances. If it is caused by an abrupt change such as acute respiratory failure the renal homeostatic mechanisms only develop fully after 3 to 5 days. A sudden acid challenge such as that following release of a tourniquet applied to the lower limb for 2 hours (e.g. orthopaedic operation under epidural anaesthesia), causes alterations in the values of the blood acid–base status that change rapidly with time as respiratory reflexes take place. Following this rapid respiratory phase over the course of a few minutes, a slower renal phase follows in the course of the next hours.

The four clinical situations described below usually progress in two phases. The initial phase is well understood and could easily be mimicked *in vitro* by adding or removing CO_2 or acid to a sample of arterial blood in a test-tube and measuring the pH and $PaCO_2$.

The compensation and compensated phase that follow the first as the homeostatic mechanisms take place, is a much more complex phenomenon that is still poorly understood. For example, the study of a sudden acid load is in some respects comparable to the study of multicompartmental kinetics of distribution and elimination of an intravenous dose of a drug (Appendix A).

(1) *Respiratory acidosis*
The commonest situation; it means retention of CO_2 due to respiratory failure or inadequate ventilation of the lungs. The causes are many, and are dealt with in Chapter 11. In acute CO_2 retention, blood [H^+] rises by about 6 $nmol\,l^{-1}$ for each kPa rise in PCO_2 (pH drops 0.1 unit per 10 mmHg CO_2 rise). In chronic retention, renal mechanisms raise plasma [HCO_3^-] sufficiently to restore pH to nearly normal values.

(2) *Metabolic acidosis*

The second commonest situation; it may appear in a variety of disease states as follows:

—Grossly uncompensated diabetes (keto-acidosis).
—Lack of oxygen delivery to tissues, as in shock or severe hypoxia.
—Loss of intestinal alkaline secretions (e.g. severe diarrhoea, fistulae).
—Transplantation of the ureters into the ileum after total cystectomy.
—Acetazolamide therapy, which impairs bicarbonate reabsorption in the kidney.
—Failure of normal homeostatic mechanisms, as in generalised renal failure or in the more rare circumstances of renal tubular failure and glomerular failure.

(3) *Respiratory alkalosis*

This is a less common situation and may be due to spontaneous hyperventilation which occurs in certain patients for unknown reasons. Respiratory alkalosis occurs commonly in mechanically ventilated patients under anaesthesia or sedation. Acutely it causes a fall in $[H^+]$ of the same proportion as for respiratory acidosis (6 nmol l^{-1} $[H^+]$ change for 1 kPa PCO_2 change).

(4) *Metabolic alkalosis*

A rare situation, that sometimes presents clinically as tetany with normal plasma calcium levels. May be due to:

Loss of acid secretions as in compulsive vomiting or in pyloric stenosis.
Excessive ingestion of alkali (overtreatment of 'indigestion'), or intravenous administration of bicarbonate (frequently seen after successful resuscitation from cardiac arrest).
Potassium depletion (extracellular alkalosis and intracellular acidosis).

Interpretation of Blood-gas Values

Blood gas results are nearly always obtained from arterial blood. In very special circum-stances mixed venous blood may also be ana-lysed to compute oxygen consumption, cardiac output or other variables.

The sample must always be heparinised by priming the dead space of the syringe (just the hub) with a 1 : 1000 solution of heparin (failure to do this results in damage to the machine taking hours of expensive labour to repair).

The interpretation of results includes examination of the acid–base status of the blood and its oxygen-carrying capacity. It must be remembered that examination of the clinical state of the patient is the most important factor in any therapeutic decision. Arterial blood measurements are only a narrow observation window of a very complex and poorly understood homeostatic system. However, following a logical routine in the examination of the results, increases the chances of a correct diagnosis.

The use of integral microcomputers in blood-gas machines will soon be extended to provide interpretation of the results as well, following the same logical steps as the clinician.

Although SI units are now officially in use, it will be found that in the great majority of establishments blood gases are still reported in pH and mmHg.

Artifacts

The blood-gas result should match the clinical assessment of the patient; a PaO_2 of 5 kPa (38 mmHg) in a conscious, non-narcotised patient without evidence of dyspnoea or central cyanosis is almost certainly artifactual. The commonest artifact is the sampling of venous blood instead of arterial, due to faulty technique of arterial puncture. Extreme values of pH or derived parameters are likely to result from mixing of the blood sample with some acidic or basic residue in the syringe. For example, if highly concentrated subcutaneous heparin solution is used to prevent sample clotting, a very acidic result may be obtained.

Samples taken from indwelling arterial catheters attached to long plastic tubes should be preceded by withdrawal of 6–8 ml of blood into another syringe to remove the priming heparinised saline. Mixing of blood with saline will give an unexpectedly low $PaCO_2$ and a low Hb (if measured). If the machine measures Hb, care should be taken to stir the sample well just prior to injection into the cuvette, to prevent the effect of sedimentation of red cells in the syringe. The Hb value measured enters many of the calculations.

The time elapsed between taking the sample and analysing it is of little importance in clinical practice. PO_2 and PCO_2 change only by about 2% of the original value if kept in a 2 ml syringe for 1 hour at room temperature. If stored in ice samples may be kept for up to 12 hours with little change in values; this precaution is only necessary for research purposes.

Diagnosis

The method used in interpretation is a matter of individual preference. Here is a suggestion:

(1) *Hydrogen ion changes*
Normal arterial blood pH is 7.4 ± 0.05 ([H^+] = 40 ± 5); it can be below that value or above it.

If the pH is below 7.35 ([H^+] > 45), there is acidaemia:

If the $PaCO_2$ is above 40 mmHg (>5.3 kPa) there is a component of respiratory acidosis.

If $PaCO_2$ is below 40 mmHg it is certain that there is metabolic acidosis.

If the pH is above 7.45 ([H^+] < 35) there is alkalaemia:

If the PCO_2 is above 40 mmHg there is metabolic alkalosis.

If below that value, there is a component of respiratory alkalosis.

The terms acidaemia and alkalaemia refer only to the status of the blood, acid or alkaline in pH. Acidosis and alkalosis refer to pathological situations resulting from a positive or negative balance of protons, where there is a change in $PaCO_2$ or HCO_3^- in an acid or alkaline direction. However, as these changes may be compensatory, they may not lead to acidaemia or alkalaemia (e.g. a diabetic with a metabolic acidosis (and acidaemia with pH of <7.1) responds with hyperventilation and a low $PaCO_2$. The latter constitutes a respiratory alkalosis, but the patient is not alkalaemic as the change is secondary.

It is not possible to quantitate precisely metabolic acidosis and alkalosis in the whole body. Clinical observation is the only reliable indicator of the severity of the situation. In the blood sample, the degree of metabolic acidaemia or alkalaemia is easily seen by looking at the base excess value: values below −12 tend to be associated with severe acidosis, needing urgent therapy, and values above +12 are usually associated with severe alkalosis.

Note that base-excess calculations depend on the concentration of haemoglobin.

(2) *Oxygen changes*
The partial pressure of oxygen in arterial blood (PaO_2) falls with age. On average, it is approximately 13 kPa (100 mmHg) in the young adult, and declines steadily to about 10 kPa (75 mmHg) at the age of 80. There is hypoxia when PaO_2 values are 2 kPa (15 mmHg) below the expected value for the patient's age.

The peripheral arterial chemoreceptors in the aortic arch and in the bifurcation of the carotid arteries are the only known oxygen sensors in the body. They are progressively stimulated by PaO_2 values below 8 kPa (60 mmHg), causing a reflex increase in ventilation. Hypoxic drive to ventilation, such as in pulmonary oedema or at altitude, usually leads to a fall in $PaCO_2$. In acute respiratory failure, hypoxia may be accompanied by CO_2 retention.

(3) *Examples*
Table 9.1 lists approximate round values to be found in the various situations mentioned above.

Treatment of Acid–base Disturbances

The cause of the acid–base disturbance must be treated and the normal respiratory and renal homeostatic mechanisms allowed to restore the balance of protons (H^+).

Only rarely is it indicated to infuse intravenously an alkali or an acid. HCl infusions in severe alkalosis have been described in a few instances, but with doubtful benefit for the clinical status of the patient.

TABLE 9.1   Approximate values in acid–base changes

	[H⁺] $nmol\,l^{-1}$	pH	PaCO₂ kPa	PaCO₂ mmHg	PaO₂ kPa	PaO₂ mmHg	[HCO₃⁻] $mmol\,l^{-1}$	BE
Normal	40	7.40	5.3	40	13	100	25	0
A	63	7.20	5.3	40	13	100	15	−15
A'	40	7.40	3.7	21	13	100	10	−15
B	63	7.20	8.0	60	8	60	28	0
B'	40	7.40	8.0	60	8	60	40	+10
C	30	7.50	3.3	25	14	105	22	0
C'	40	7.40	3.3	25	14	105	17	−10
D	30	7.50	5.3	40	13	100	30	+10
D'	40	7.40	6.7	50	9	68	35	+10

Before any compensatory mechanism   After full compensation
A—metabolic acidosis   A'
B—respiratory acidosis   B'
C—respiratory alkalosis   C'
D—metabolic alkalosis   D'

Note that full compensation values (rarely achieved) are only of theoretical interest to indicate the direction of change. Hb = 15 g dl⁻¹.

On the other hand, sodium bicarbonate infusions have been widely employed in the past to treat severe metabolic acidosis; presently their indication has been much restricted as more deleterious side effects have been found. Its use in diabetic acidosis has practically been abandoned, and the value of its routine infusion in cardiac arrest is now in question.

Sodium bicarbonate carries a considerable load of sodium (1 mmol Na per mmol HCO₃). In addition, high CO_2 pressures are generated on mixing with acidic blood which cause diffusion of CO_2 into cells and intracellular acidosis (this is more likely in mechanically ventilated patients or those in respiratory failure, who are unable to eliminate the excess CO_2 in the first passage through the lung).

When sodium bicarbonate is considered necessary to correct acidosis, it should be remembered that the figure for base excess refers to the deficit of bicarbonate in the extracellular fluid (ECF). Thus, it is necessary to calculate ECF in litres and multiply this by the BE to arrive at a figure for sodium bicarbonate in mmol. In adults, about ⅓ to ⅕ of body weight is ECF, whilst in babies it is about ⅖. Usually only ½ the calculated amount is given initially, e.g.

Weight = 60 kg
BE   = −12
ECF   = 0.3 × 60 = 18 litres

Thus,

NaHCO₃   needed = 18 × 12 = 216 mmol   (half this amount initially)

NB. Sodium bicarbonate must never be given if PaCO₂ is raised or there is any evidence that the patient has respiratory impairment, as the CO_2 generated by the reaction of fixed acid with sodium bicarbonate must be cleared by the lungs.

Arterial Puncture

Only arterial puncture for sampling of blood for gas measurement will be discussed. Arterial

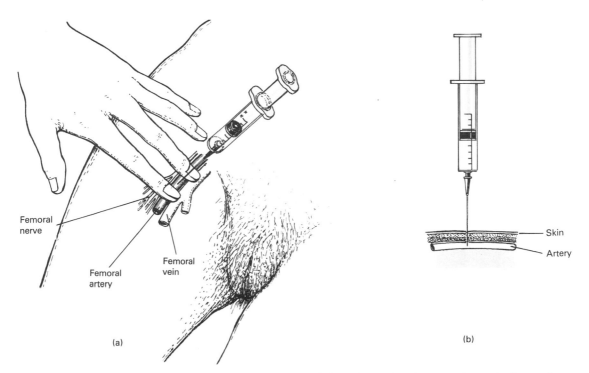

Fig. 9.3 Arterial puncture. (a) Position of the fingers of the left hand, palpating the right femoral artery. (b) Position of the needle relative to the skin

cannulation is a more specialised manoeuvre outside the scope of this book.

With very rare exceptions, only the radial and femoral arteries should be used for this purpose. The volume of blood required for gas and acid–base balance measurements is only 0.5 ml so a 1 ml sample carried in a 2 ml syringe is plenty. It should be taken with the smallest diameter needle allowing a rapid flow of blood into the syringe, i.e. 23G (blue hub), to minimise damage to the arterial wall.

Firstly, the dead space of the syringe must be filled with a 1:1000 solution of heparin and all the air removed; the needle must be firmly attached to the hub so air is not drawn in on suctioning. Both radial and femoral artery are more easily punctured by introducing the needle perpendicular to the skin (Fig. 9.3).

In the femoral, the second and third fingers of the left hand should be kept over the course of the artery and the pulsation felt in both fingers which are kept some 1 cm apart. The needle is then inserted in between the two fingers applying a gentle constant pull to the plunger of the syringe; on entering the arterial lumen a sudden 'give' is usually felt and blood appears in the syringe.

In the radial artery the following alternative technique may be more effective: extend the wrist joint and start by feeling the arterial pulse with one finger some 2 cm proximal to the wrist, and mark the point where it is felt with a dot, using an ordinary pen. Repeat this procedure 2 or 3 times at steps 5 mm proximally to the last point; this way the course of the artery is identified by doing a mental 'curve fitting' exercise. Then, keeping the wrist extended insert the needle into the artery following the same procedure as for the femoral.

There are specially made syringes for blood-gas sampling which are previously heparinised and allow the blood to flow in by its own pressure, avoiding the accidental sampling of venous blood.

If it is suspected that the needle has entered a vein then the syringe may be disconnected from the needle and the absence of brisk blood flow through the latter confirms venous puncture.

10

Mechanical ventilation and ventilators

Indications

Apart from the common requirement to ventilate patients during surgery (Chapter 1) mechanical ventilation (intermittent positive pressure ventilation, IPPV) is needed in any case of respiratory failure which has proceeded, despite treatment, to the point at which either oxygen administration by mask is insufficient to correct severe hypoxaemia or carbon dioxide retention has rapidly reached dangerous levels (e.g. $PaO_2 < 6$ kPa or 45 mmHg, $PaCO_2 > 9$ kPa or 70 mmHg). Less well-defined criteria for IPPV include; following major surgery (e.g. cardiac or neurological) or trauma, where IPPV is continued post-operatively until vital parameters such as temperature, haemoglobin, electrolytes and cardiac function have returned to normal. Some patients may need IPPV on clinical grounds of distress or exhaustion, despite maintenance of relatively normal blood gases.

Technique

(a) Setting up

Institution of IPPV often occurs in circumstances which are far from controlled, so preferably a special 'intubating' cart should be available at all times. The 'MS MAID' mnemonic is useful if such a cart is not to hand. 'M' stands for anaesthetic machine, and includes a source of pressurised oxygen (O_2); 'S' stands for suction apparatus which works and can reach the patient; 'M' stands for monitoring of pulse, blood pressure

and ECG; 'A' stands for airway equipment such as reservoir bag, face mask, oral airway, endotracheal tubes, laryngoscopes and syringe for cuff inflation; 'I' stands for intravenous access and finally 'D' stands for all the drugs likely to be necessary such as atropine, intravenous induction agents, opiates, neuromuscular blocking drugs and so on. Finally, skilled assistance is of vital importance.

(b) The patient

Inform the patient (if conscious) and the relatives of what is happening and its implications, e.g. patient will be sedated and unable to communicate.

(c) Intubation

Proceed to intubate with general or local anaesthesia. Following intubation, ensure correct placement of tube (e.g. inspection of chest movement, auscultation of breath sounds and chest X-ray, Chapter 4).

(d) Ventilator

Set up the ventilator and start IPPV. Ventilators vary but in all cases a predicted minute volume and fraction of inspired oxygen (FIO_2) must be calculated (e.g. minute volume of 100 ml kg^{-1} min^{-1} respiratory frequency 10 bpm, FIO_2 0.4). This must be confirmed by frequent measurement of expired volumes and checking of FIO_2 with a polarographic or fuel cell oxygen analyser; adequacy of the settings should be checked by frequent measurement of arterial blood gases. It is important that severe hypercapnoea (i.e. $CO_2 > 10$ kPa or 80 mmHg) is not corrected too suddenly as this may be associated with profound cardiovascular depression.

Pathophysiological Effects of IPPV

(a) Cardiac

The positive intrathoracic pressure (versus the normal negative) means that venous return to the heart is impeded, this together with compression tamponade tends to lower cardiac output. This is exacerbated by the addition of positive end expiratory pressure (PEEP). Institution of IPPV and intubation with depressant drugs is often associated with hypotension for this reason. In most cases, correction of a low (<5 cm H_2O) central venous pressure with administration of appropriate fluids restores blood pressure (and cardiac output). In exceptional cases, persistent hypotension, despite a reasonable CVP, demands the insertion of a pulmonary artery catheter, assessment and optimisation of pulmonary capillary wedge pressure (PCWP) with addition of inotropes as required (Chapter 14).

(b) Pulmonary

Although collapsed alveoli are re-expanded by IPPV and PEEP, normal alveoli may be subjected to very high inflation pressures and can suffer barotrauma with rupture leading to pneumothorax. IPPV with regular, unchanging tidal volumes eventually leads to atelectasis, so regular chest physiotherapy is mandatory. This involves regular inflation of the patient's chest with large tidal volumes together with endotracheal suction of secretions. Some ventilators can be set to mimic the normal physiological mechanism for prevention of atelectasis, i.e. 'sighing', by intermittent administration of large volumes (1 to 2 litres) which interpose the regular unchanging mechanical breaths.

(c) Splanchnic

Interference with venous return may decrease liver, kidney and gut blood flow leading to defective function of these organs.

(d) Other

Intubation bypasses the humidifying and bactericidal upper respiratory tract, therefore artificial humidification is necessary, together with scrupulous asepsis.

Mechanical Ventilators

These are mechanical devices, driven by electrical power or compressed gas source, which mimic normal respiratory patterns except that the air/oxygen mixture is under positive pressure. Modern machines may be incredibly sophisticated and include onboard microcomputers with push button control of tidal volume, respiratory frequency, inspired oxygen concentration and so on. All provide the following four phases:

(a) Inspiratory phase

The motive power may be either by pressure generation (e.g. weight on a bellows) or flow generation (e.g. piston controlled by a reciprocating motor). The pressure that can be obtained is usually limited to about 6 kPa or 60 cmH₂O to minimise the risk of barotrauma, but this pressure may have to be exceeded with asthmatics (Chapter 11).

(b) Cycling from inspiration to expiration

After the requisite tidal volume has entered the patient, the ventilator must stop and cycle to expiration. This is achieved by time, volume or pressure cycling. This means that the switching over from inspiration to expiration can be actuated by a device triggered by a pre-set time, volume or pressure respectively.

(c) Expiratory phase

If respiratory frequency is 10 bpm (cycle = 6 s), inspiration takes 2 seconds, then the ventilator must open to the atmosphere for 4 seconds to allow gas to leave the lungs by elastic recoil. In many ventilators there is a one-way valve on the expiratory limb, so that if the patient tries to take a breath, negative pressure is generated and no air enters the lungs. In the technique of intermittent mandatory ventilation (IMV) a separate flow of gas is made available for the patient to breathe. This allows for the ventilator rate to be gradually reduced so that the patient progressively takes over the work of breathing. Also, during expiration, a backpressure may be applied to provide PEEP.

(d) Cycling from expiration to inspiration

Finally, after 4 seconds of expiration, the ventilator must switch back to inspiration for the cycle to be repeated. This is usually time cycled.

(e) PEEP and CPAP

PEEP means maintaining the pressure in the lung above atmospheric during the whole of expiration. Normally, in IPPV the expired gas passes into the atmosphere without any obstruction to flow. With PEEP a precisely regulated resistance to expiratory flow is inserted into the ventilator, such that expiratory pressures are maintained at values set between 0 and 20 cm of water.

PEEP is indicated when there is hypoxia due to a reduced functional residual capacity (FRC) with small airway closure. It can cause a dramatic improvement in the oxygenation of the blood by increasing FRC without the necessity to utilise toxic concentrations of oxygen (Chapter 12).

CPAP stands for continuous positive airway pressure, and is applied to patients breathing spontaneously. The indications are the same as for PEEP.

Weaning from IPPV

One of the most difficult problems is the assessment of when the patient no longer needs respiratory assistance. In many cases, such as postoperative or short-term IPPV of less than 24 hours, IPPV is discontinued abruptly and the endotracheal tube removed shortly thereafter. However, after protracted periods of IPPV this is not possible, so it is important to assess firstly, the patient's overall status with regard to awareness and response, peripheral circulation, blood pressure, paralysis and sedation and, secondly, to assess the probability that the respiratory apparatus (lung, muscles and chest wall) will be able to perform adequate gaseous exchange. The latter is often 'hit and miss' but certain guidelines can be laid down:

(a) Arterial blood gases

Before considering the withdrawal of ventilatory support, the PaO_2 should be >8 kPa (60 mmHg) and $PaCO_2$ < 6.7 kPa (50 mmHg) with reasonable FIO_2 (<0.6), minute volume (<150 ml kg^{-1}) and PEEP < 0.5 kPa (5 cmH$_2$O), from the machine.

(b) Forced vital capacity (FVC)

If the above criteria are met, the patient is disconnected from the machine, a spirometer is inserted into the catheter mount and the patient requested to take as big a breath in as possible and then to breathe out for as long as possible. FVC should exceed 15 ml kg^{-1} for weaning to be successful.

If satisfactory, the patient is disconnected from the machine for 15 minutes every hour and according to the clinical status and arterial blood gases, this period is extended until eventually IPPV is no longer required. The patient is then extubated.

In more difficult cases, particularly those requiring PEEP, a more gradual process is adopted as mentioned above under IMV. The contribution of the ventilator is gradually reduced to about 2 breaths/minute and then the patient is allowed to breathe entirely on his own. The patient is then extubated provided 'normal' blood gases (see above) are maintained. Repeated attempts may be necessary, and if the period of IPPV exceeds 10 days, a tracheostomy is performed, which may make weaning easier and more comfortable for the patient.

Physiological Effects of Alteration in Arterial Carbon Dioxide as a Result of IPPV. Determination of Ventilator Settings

(a) Effects of alteration in $PaCO_2$

CO_2 retention is such a common finding that there has been a tendency to ignore the effects of an acute reduction, especially during IPPV. Lack of monitoring (end tidal CO_2, or blood gases) during balanced relaxant anaesthesia often leads to very low arterial carbon dioxide tensions ($PaCO_2$), and this may have serious adverse effects:

1 Respiratory alkalosis resulting in post-operative hypoventilation and consequent hypoxia
2 A left shift in the oxygen dissociation curve (decreased p50), thus increasing haemoglobin oxygen affinity and decreasing release of oxygen to the tissues (Chapter 12)
3 A decrease in ionised calcium leading to decreased myocardial contractility
4 A decreased cerebral blood flow (of which $PaCO_2$ is a major determinant). Although this is used therapeutically to reduce raised intracranial pressure, it can cause stagnant cerebral hypoxia in the elderly, especially if anaemic
5 a decreased coronary blood flow which can prejudice the oxygen supply/demand ratio of the myocardium

In general, raising the $PaCO_2$ has opposite effects to the above (Chapter 11). Thus it should be noted that gross alteration in $PaCO_2$ up or down can have deleterious effects in some patients.

(b) Factors to consider for maintaining normocapnoea during IPPV

Arterial carbon dioxide tension is determined by two factors:

CO_2 production ($\dot{V}_{CO_2}$)
CO_2 elimination (alveolar ventilation, $\dot{V}_A$)

i.e. $PaCO_2 = (\dot{V}_{CO_2})/\dot{V}_A$, over the normal clinical range (Chapter 9)

Normally,

$$(\dot{V}_{CO_2}) = 200 \text{ ml min} \quad (\text{roughly } 3 \text{ ml kg}^{-1})$$
$$\dot{V}_A = 5 \text{ l min}^{-1}$$

Thus,
$$PaCO_2 = 200/5$$
$$= 40 \text{ mmHg (5.3 kPa)}$$

(1) $\dot{V}_{CO_2}$

This is roughly 3 ml kg^{-1} body weight, being slightly higher in the infant and slightly lower in the elderly. It increases with metabolic rate by about 20–30% per °C increase, and declines by about the same amount with decreases in body temperature. During anaesthesia, it is reduced by about 10% from the normal value.

(2) $\dot{V}_A$

Ventilators are set to deliver a minute volume (MV) to the patient, this being the product of respiratory frequency (RF) and tidal volume (V_T). However, some of the ventilation is wasted due to 'dead space' (V_D).

Thus $\dot{V}_A = (V_T - V_D) \times RF$

V_D includes both the air passages (anatomical dead space) and regions of the lung where ventilation exceeds perfusion (alveolar dead space, $\dot{V}/\dot{Q} > 1$). It is best considered as a fraction of V_T, normally it is 0.3. Thus, a minute volume of about 7 l min^{-1} is needed to get an alveolar ventilation of 5 l min^{-1}.

Example:

A 70 kg male has an estimated ($\dot{V}_{CO_2}$) of $70 \times 3 = 210 \text{ ml min}^{-1}$: To achieve a $PaCO_2$ of 40 mmHg (5.3 kPa) he will need an alveolar ventilation of

$5\,l\,min^{-1}$ which with a V_D/V_T of 0.3 necessitates a minute volume of $7\,l\,min^{-1}$ $(100\,ml\,kg^{-1}\,min^{-1})$. This is the same as the figure mentioned earlier, and it should now be more clear as to how this value is derived. In practice, the reduction in metabolic rate during anaesthesia usually results in the patient having a slightly lower $PaCO_2$ than normal.

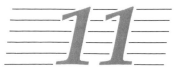

Respiratory emergencies

Definition

Acute respiratory failure (ARF) exists when the patient's breathing apparatus fails in its ability to maintain arterial blood gases within the normal range. By definition, ARF is present when the blood gases demonstrate:

An arterial oxygen tension (PaO_2) of <8 kPa (60 mmHg) and/or

An arterial carbon dioxide tension ($PaCO_2$) of >6.7 kPa (50 mmHg)

These are usually accompanied by a fall in pH (<7.3, $H^+ > 45$ n mols l^{-1})

Pathophysiology

Any part of the respiratory apparatus may be involved in the causation of a respiratory emergency, from the central nervous system (CNS) to the alveoli. Examples are shown in Table 11.1.

Clinical Picture

The clinical picture varies with the cause but any of those mentioned in Table 11.1 leads to a deterioration in the patient's respiratory gas exchange. The subsequent changes which occur in blood gases, particularly carbon dioxide, cause stimulation of the medullary chemoreceptor and compensatory mechanisms to be activated. The patient becomes aware of the necessity to breathe, and as the precipitating cause progresses, exhibits overt signs of distress, i.e. dyspnoea. Eventually blood gases can no longer be kept in the normal range and ARF supervenes.

ARF resulting from CNS depression as a result

TABLE 11.1

Site	Examples
CNS	Depressant drugs, opiates; traumatic and ischaemic lesions
Peripheral nerves	Guillain Barré, poliomyelitis
Neuromuscular junction	Myasthenia, neuromuscular blocking drugs
Muscle	Myopathies, respiratory muscle fatigue
Airways	Extrathoracic: foreign bodies, croup Intrathoracic: asthma, bronchiolitis, bronchitis
Gaseous exchange	Emphysema, pulmonary oedema, ARDS, pneumonia
Lung vasculature Pleura and thoracic cage	Pulmonary embolus, ARDS, Flail chest, pneumothorax, haemothorax

ARDS refers to adult respiratory distress syndrome.

of drugs or injury does not produce overt signs of respiratory distress. Accurate diagnosis is dependent on a high index of suspicion and is confirmed by arterial blood gas analysis.

Signs of acute respiratory failure of peripheral origin

Generally, the onset of ARF is heralded by the patient becoming anxious and completely preoccupied with the necessity to concentrate every effort on ventilation. The eyes are closed, the accessory muscles of ventilation are fully used; often a characteristic position is adopted, such as sitting forward with drooling secretions, as in the child with acute epiglottitis. Hypoxia and hypercarbia produce characteristic effects on the CNS and cardiovascular system (CVS), for example:

1 Hypoxia: CNS – Uncooperative, confused, drunken-like state
              CVS – Bradycardia, variable blood pressure, cyanosis

2 Hypercarbia: CNS – Tremor and overt flap
                CVS – Raised pulse rate, peripheral vasodilatation with pink peripheries, blood pressure changes are variable

Diagnosis

Diagnosis depends on history, clinical examination and special investigations such as chest X-ray, peak expiratory flow rate and arterial blood gas analysis. It is important to establish the causative site (Table 11.1).

For example, the history gives a clue to pre-existing disease such as chronic bronchitis and asthma, or may distinguish between acute epiglottitis (sudden onset) and laryngotracheobronchitis (slower onset over 24 hours), when the clinical signs are equivocal. On clinical examination, expiratory wheeze suggests intrathoracic airway obstruction whilst inspiratory wheeze suggests that it is extrathoracic. Chest X-ray will reveal parenchymal causes such as pneumonia, airway obstruction due to foreign bodies (ipsilateral hyperinflation of lung), pleural and thoracic cage causes, such as effusion, pneumothorax and fractured ribs. Raised bicarbonate levels in the blood gases suggest chronic pre-existing disease, and a combination of hypoxia, hypocarbia and an initial metabolic alkalosis followed by acidosis is a common accompaniment of ARDS.

Treatment

Whatever the cause, four important principles of treatment apply:

(a) Establish an airway

This applies particularly to the unconscious patient, e.g. due to overdose, general anaesthesia, CNS trauma and so on. The patient is placed on the side with the head down, and lower jaw pulled forward to prevent the tongue falling back and obstructing the upper airway. At this stage it may become obvious that the obstruction is due primarily to foreign bodies or vomit, so this must be cleared, if possible.

(1) *Indications for artificial airways*
Oropharyngeal: this is useful where it is expected that the patient will soon recover consciousness, e.g. post-operatively, or where there is lack of expertise in endotracheal intubation.

(2) *Endotracheal tube (ETT)*
If unconsciousness is expected to last for more than a matter of minutes, as in drug overdose, then an ETT must be used both to ensure and to protect the airway (e.g. from aspiration of gastric contents). If ventilation is depressed or inadequate due to trauma or disease, then mechanical ventilation will be required.

(3) *Cricothyrotomy and tracheotomy*
Obstruction above the cords due to disease or infection may make intubation impossible. Cricothyrotomy or tracheotomy is then necessary to restore the airway (Chapter 4).

(b) Administer oxygen to ensure adequate tissue oxygenation

It is of paramount importance to maintain a PaO_2 sufficient to give an arterial Hb saturation of at least 85% (i.e. 8–9 kPa or 60–70 mmHg). Hyperoxia should be avoided, particularly in the bronchitic who is a CO_2 retainer and dependent on hypoxic ventilatory drive.

(c) Maintain alveolar ventilation and treat underlying cause

These two are inextricably linked. The causes of acute respiratory failure are many and varied as are the requisite therapies. If treatment of the underlying cause is not successful (i.e. steroids, bronchodilators in asthma; physiotherapy, antibiotics, mucolytics, bronchodilators in acute on chronic bronchitis), then the carbon dioxide tension will begin to rise, necessitating intermittent positive pressure ventilation (IPPV). There is little place for respiratory stimulants, except perhaps narcotic antagonists in opiate overdose.

Special Problems Encountered in the Intensive Care Unit (ICU)

Despite the fact that there are many causes of ARF, anaesthetists in ICU are faced with a relatively small number of problems which occur frequently:

(a) The croup syndrome

Upper airway obstruction in the small child represents one of the most life-threatening situations in clinical medicine. Croup means literally 'noisy breathing' and is due to upper airway obstruction, conventionally delineated into supra- and subglottic. The most common causes are infectious and traumatic.

(1) *Infectious*

Supraglottic obstruction is usually due to epiglottitis. The main features of the disease are rapid onset of severe respiratory obstruction and a high temperature with the patient adopting the classical sitting position with drooling secretions.

The diagnosis is made on the history and clinical findings, and as the child (usually 3 to 7 years old) may completely obstruct at any time, he or she must be taken immediately to the operating theatre with an experienced anaesthetist and surgeon prepared for endotracheal intubation (ETI) or tracheotomy. This is usually performed under general anaesthesia as attempted manipulations to visualise the epiglottis in the awake patient often results in total obstruction and death. Following preferably nasotracheal intubation, the child is sedated and treated for *Haemophilus influenzae* infection with ampicillin and other appropriate antibiotics together with humidification of inspired gases.

Subglottic obstruction is usually due to laryngotracheobronchitis, with a much more slowly progressive course, lower temperature and fewer signs of respiratory obstruction. Intubation is required more rarely, and less often in a hurry. However, the clinical course is often more protracted and, once instituted, ETI is needed for longer periods than with epiglottitis.

(2) *Trauma*

This may be due to instrumentation (e.g. post-extubation), inhalation of a foreign body, external trauma or aspiration of noxious substances such as acid or alkali. The history will usually confirm the diagnosis. Treatment will depend on the cause, but usually requires intubation and steroid administration, and in the case of foreign body, operative removal with bronchoscopy.

(b) Acute (status) asthma

By the time the patient with an acute asthmatic attack reaches the ICU, the anaesthetist is faced with one of the most difficult managment problems. The patient is often exhausted, tachycardic, hypoxic, hypercarbic, acidotic and dehydrated, yet needs intubation and ventilation to restore reasonable blood gases. Attempting to intubate the patient 'awake' may precipitate 'terminal' bronchospasm, yet even the administration of the most gentle anaesthetic may precipitate cardiovascular collapse. Following intubation, ventilation is usually extremely difficult necessitating high inflation pressures which can only be lowered by prolonging inspiration, and yet air trapping requires that expiration is also prolonged. This conundrum requires considerable compromise with ventilator settings and can often only be accommodated by accepting relatively high $PaCO_2$ levels.

(c) The chronic bronchitic requiring ventilation

In a previous section it was mentioned that the chronic bronchitic who presents in ARF may proceed, despite optimal therapy, to the point where intubation and ventilation (IPPV) is required. In such cases it is paramount that the patient is assessed as to the suitability of this form of treatment. This involves a thorough history from the patient (or relatives) with particular regard to:

Previous hospital admissions, with lung function tests and blood gases
Previous requirements for IPPV or tracheostomy
Exercise tolerance

Only guidelines can be given, but in cases where the patient has had frequent previous admissions with IPPV treatment, progressive lung damage can be anticipated so that further periods of IPPV may be unwarranted. This is also applicable to cases where the patient is housebound and/or breathless at rest. If IPPV is instituted in such cases weaning from IPPV may be impossible (Chapter 10).

(d) Adult Respiratory Distress Syndrome (ARDS)

In recent years, it has become evident that the lung can be injured as a secondary process in severe illness or trauma. Generally speaking it is the vascular endothelium (either bronchial venular or capillary) which is affected. Damage from any of the causes below results in loss of membrane integrity and thus increased permeability to fluid and protein. This leaks into the interstitial space and lymphatics, producing 'non-cardiogenic pulmonary oedema', with a characteristic 'fluffy' appearance on chest X-ray.

It is distinguished from 'cardiogenic pulmonary oedema', by demonstration of a normal or low pulmonary capillary wedge pressure, and from oedema due to a low colloid oncotic pressure by demonstration of a serum albumin of $>30\,g\,l^{-1}$. A pronounced decrease in functional residual capacity (FRC) and compliance occurs, with a resulting increased work of breathing and dyspnoea. This together with the associated vascular damage results in an imbalance of ventilation and perfusion, with hypoxia and increase in dead space. ARDS may result from:

1 ischaemia (following major trauma and hypotension),
2 complement and neutrophil activation (as in sepsis, or prolonged hypovolaemia)
3 disseminated intravascular coagulation (DIC) with vascular microthrombosis and ischaemia
4 fat embolus syndrome
5 acid aspiration causes primarily alveolar epithelial damage, but vascular endothelial damage follows leading to ARDS
6 inhalation injury, e.g. noxious fumes

The symptoms are those of severe ARF with dyspnoea being prominent. The 'clinical' condition of the patient may not immediately give cause for concern, e.g. in early 'fat embolism'. However, sampling of the arterial blood gases reveals profound hypoxaemia ($PaO_2 < 5\,kPa$ or $35\,mmHg$) and secondary hyperventilation with a low $PaCO_2$ ($<4\,kP$ or $30\,mmHg$). If left untreated, CO_2 retention and metabolic acidosis develop. The profound hypoxia is often unresponsive to additional oxygen by mask, in which case ETI with IPPV and positive end expiratory pressure (PEEP) is required. The latter works by increasing FRC by backward distending pressure thus reducing $\dot{V}/\dot{Q}$ mismatch and improving compliance at the same time.

12

Oxygen therapy and oxygen toxicity

Introduction

Oxygen is essential to life due to its function as the final electron and H^+ acceptor in the mitochondrial cytochrome chain whereby ATP is produced as the cellular energy source. Without 'aerobic' metabolism, ATP production is not only reduced 20-fold but lactic acid is produced in excess, causing intracellular acidosis and eventually death. The reserves of ATP are small, so a constant supply of oxygen is necessary for living cells. Many disease states lead to failure to deliver oxygen to tissues, which often is the ultimate cause of death. Also, following anaesthesia and surgery, oxygen delivery is usually compromised at various levels.

(a) The patient's respiratory drive is diminished as a result of opiate analgesics and residual quantities of other central nervous system (CNS) depressants.

(b) When controlled ventilation is instituted during balanced anaesthesia there is often a tendency to reduce the patient's arterial carbon dioxide tension ($PaCO_2$). This, together with the effect of residual CNS depressants, leads to hypoventilation in the immediate post-operative period until $PaCO_2$ has been restored to normality. During this period, oxygen delivery may be insufficient to maintain oxygenation unless its concentration in the inspired gas is increased.

(c) The capacity to ventilate the lungs and to cough may also be impaired due to residual effects of long-acting neuromuscular blockers and to pain.

(d) The metabolic demand for oxygen may be increased by temperature, and the oxygen-carrying capacity of blood decreased due to red cell loss.

(e) A cold operating theatre, administration of inadequately warmed fluids and blood, lack of warming and humidification of inspired gases, loss of the patient's normal mechanisms of heat conservation under anaesthesia (Chapter 15), exposure of large areas of bowel and so on all contribute to loss of heat and reduction of body temperature during major surgery. As soon as the operation is complete, the patient restores body temperature to normal by shivering, resulting in big increases in oxygen demand.

(f) If the cardiac output is significantly reduced due to heart disease or to depressant drugs, regional perfusion is impaired as well.

These are some of the important reasons why oxygen therapy is indicated post-operatively.

Blood Oxygen Content and Dissociation Curve

Haemoglobin is employed as a specialised oxygen carrying system. Simple solution of oxygen in plasma, at ambient pressure and concentration, is insufficient for cellular oxygen demand (0.3 ml of O_2 per 100 ml of plasma). The relation between the partial pressure of oxygen in blood and haemoglobin saturation is a sigmoid curve, with the steepest portion occurring

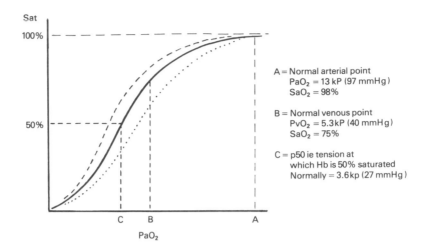

Fig. 12.1 The haemoglobin dissociation curve.
..... = R shift due to increase in CO_2, H^+, temperature, 2, 3dpg*
(increased p50).
----- = L shift due to decrease in CO_2, H^+, temperature, 2, 3dpg
(decreased p50).
*2, 3dpg – is formed from 1, 3dpg in the glycolytic pathway. It
binds preferentially to the reduced form of Hb thereby aiding O_2
release to the tissues.

in the range 2.6–9.3 kPa (20–70 mmHg) as seen
in Fig. 12.1. One gram of haemoglobin can carry
1.34 ml of oxygen when fully saturated. Thus
with a Hb of 15 g dl^{-1}, an arterial oxygen tension
(PaO_2) of 13.3 kPa (100 mmHg) and a saturation
(SaO_2) of 98%:

Arterial oxygen content:

$= 15 \times 1.34 \times 0.98$
$= 20$ ml 100 ml^{-1} of blood (ignore that dis-
solved in plasma)
$= 200$ ml l^{-1}

Oxygen Cascade from Environment to Cell

Oxygen therapy is ultimately designed to ensure
adequate mitochondrial oxygen tensions. The
points at which failure to achieve this may occur
are outlined in Table 12.1.

(a) Oxygen consumption

As oxygen is taken up from alveolus to capillary,
its partial pressure in the alveolus (PAO_2)
declines unless oxygen is constantly added by
ventilation. At a normal oxygen consumption of
250 ml min^{-1} with alveolar ventilation of
5 l min^{-1}, the PAO_2 is 13.3 kPa (100 mmHg). If
oxygen consumption doubles, as a result of raised temperature, excessive muscular activity or
shivering, then the same alveolar ventilation
only results in a PAO_2 of 8 kPa (60 mmHg).
Although the healthy patient may be able to
double or treble alveolar ventilation to com-
pensate for the increased demand, post-operative or sick patients may not. Increasing the
inspired oxygen fraction (FIO_2) to 0.4 partially
compensates.

(b) Arterial blood

Ventilation ($\dot{V}$) and perfusion ($\dot{Q}$) must be

TABLE 12.1 Causes and classification of hypoxia

System level	Defect	Classification
1 Inspired gas	Inspired oxygen tension (PIO_2)	Hypoxic
	Low barometric pressure (pB)	Hypoxic
2 Inspired gas to alveolar gas	(a) Low alveolar ventilation	Hypoxic
	(b) Raised oxygen consumption	Hypoxic
3 Alveolar gas to arterial blood	(a) Venous admixture or shunt	Hypoxic
	(b) $\dot{V}/\dot{Q}$ scatter (>1)	Hypoxic
4 Arterial blood to cell	(a) Low or inadequate blood flow	Stagnant
		Anaemic
	(b) Low Hb	Anaemic
	(c) Carbon monoxide poisoning	
5 Cell	Metabolic poisons	Histotoxic

closely matched so that oxygen delivery by ventilation to the lungs ($1000\,ml\,min^{-1}$) matches oxygen uptake and transport from the lungs to the tissues ($1000\,ml\,min^{-1}$). Although we can look at the lung as a whole, it is obviously important that each alveolus and its perfusing blood supply are also closely matched for V and Q in a ratio of 1:1. In health, due to the effect of gravity, the alveoli at the base of the lung tend to be relatively overperfused (V/Q 0.8:1) whilst those at the apex which do not receive such a good blood supply are relatively over ventilated (V/Q 2:1). Overall, the figure is close to 0.9:1.

If ventilation to an alveolus is restricted (due to collapse, atelectasis and so on) and its perfusion maintained, then the V/Q ratio would fall from around 1:1 to say 0.2:1. Oxygen uptake exceeds supply so the blood leaving the alveolus is not properly oxygenated. This hypoxic blood meets arterialised blood from normal alveoli and results in an overall reduction of PaO_2. This is called 'venous admixture' and is correctable by increasing the FIO_2. This has the effect of increasing the actual amount of oxygen reaching the alveolus by increasing the concentration.

If ventilation to an alveolus is obstructed completely, no amount of additional oxygen will help and the patient has a true 'shunt'. This may be due to complete atelectasis or an extrapulmonary shunt as in congenital heart disease.

Therapeutic implications

Although simply increasing the FIO_2 counteracts the deleterious effects of atelectasis in the short term, no effort should be spared in assisting the patient to re-expand the collapsed alveoli. Atelectasis, due to inadequate ventilation, predisposes to infection and effectively reduces lung volume and respiratory reserve. Thus, especially following upper abdominal surgery, and particularly if the patient is a heavy smoker or has chronic obstructive pulmonary disease, breathing exercises and physiotherapy are encouraged to prevent this serious complication.

(c) Oxygen delivery to cells

Oxygen carried in blood leaving the lungs has to reach the cells to allow aerobic metabolism to take place. The concept of tissue 'oxygen delivery' or 'availability' is an important one because it gives a good idea of the factors determining tissue oxygenation.

Oxygen delivery = arterial oxygen content × cardiac output (see above)

Normally, cardiac output (Q) is about $5\,l\,min^{-1}$

$$Oxygen\ delivery = 200 \times 5$$
$$= 1000\,ml\,min^{-1}$$

Note the three variables which affect oxygen availability; Hb, SaO_2 and Q. At an oxygen consumption of $250\,ml\,min^{-1}$, this leaves 750 ml of oxygen returning to the lung in the venous blood. If each one of the variables is halved, oxygen delivery is reduced to $\frac{1}{8}$ of normal, $125\,ml\,min^{-1}$. This results in anaerobic metabolism, lactic acid production and cellular acidosis.

Types of Hypoxia

(a) Anoxic or hypoxic

This is due to a fall in the partial pressure of the inspired gas (PIO_2) such as at altitude, or if inspired oxygen is reduced in accidental misconnection of pipes under anaesthesia. This results in a fall in PAO_2. An increase in $PaCO_2$ or in the alveolar to arterial gradient for oxygen $((A\text{-}a)dO_2)$ lowers PaO_2 directly.

(b) Anaemic

This is due to failure of oxygen carriage, as a result of low Hb, with normal cardiac output and saturation, or to alteration in the oxygen carrying capacity of Hb as a result of combination with carbon monoxide. The latter binds more strongly to Hb than does oxygen with the result that the tissues receive an inadequate oxygen supply.

(c) Stagnant or ischaemic

This results from inadequate blood perfusion to tissues due to myocardial failure, sepsis, raised systemic vascular resistance, or arterial embolism.

(d) Histotoxic

Here the oxygen delivery to the tissues is normal, but mitochondrial oxygen utilisation is defective, such as in cyanide poisoning.

Oxygen Administration

From the above, it can be seen that raising the FIO_2 is a primary form of treatment for many of the conditions causing hypoxia. It is symptomatic and not curative.

The effect that increased FIO_2 has on PAO_2 can be determined from the 'alveolar air equation', i.e.

$$PAO_2 = PIO_2 - PaCO_2/R$$

PIO_2 refers to the inspired O_2 tension ($FIO_2 \times$ barometric pressure, BP). Thus at an FIO_2 of 0.4, and a BP of 713 (760 mmHg − water vapour pressure in the lungs of 47 mmHg), PIO_2 is equal to about 280. R refers to the respiratory exchange ratio, i.e. the amount of CO_2 produced divided by the amount of O_2 consumed (in ml min^{-1}). This ratio is normally 0.8. Thus if the PIO_2 is 280 and $PaCO_2$ is 40,

$$PAO_2 = 280 - 40/0.8$$
$$= 230$$

The difference between the calculated PAO_2 and the actual PaO_2 gives the 'A-a' gradient, $(A\text{-}a)dO_2$. This is a useful estimate of the amount of venous admixture or shunted blood passing through the lungs without coming into contact with alveolar air. An increase in the gradient suggests an increased shunt. The alveolar air equation also emphasises the deleterious effect on PaO_2 of a rise in $PaCO_2$, and why an increase in FIO_2 goes some way in compensation.

Devices for delivering oxygen (raising the FIO_2) include masks, nasal prongs, tents and hyperbaric chambers.

Types of device

Two types are in common use:

(1) *Low flow devices*

These are simple, cheap devices such as the Mary Catterall (MC), Hudson mask and nasal prongs. A fixed flow of oxygen (2–4 l min^{-1}) enters the mask (or nasopharynx) so that the patient inspires an oxygen–air mixture. The flow of oxygen is less than the air flow during inspiration so the final oxygen concentration is determined, not only by the oxygen flow rate into the mask but also by the patient's minute volume. If the latter declines, the fractional concentration of inspired oxygen (FIO_2) increases. In those patients dependent on hypoxic drive with chronic CO_2 retention, too high an initial FIO_2 may be achieved, leading to hyperoxia, hypoventilation and a further rise in FIO_2 as the minute volume falls. The ensuing increase in $PaCO_2$ may be sufficient to render the patient unconscious.

For this reason, low flow devices are reserved for those patients in whom a precise knowledge

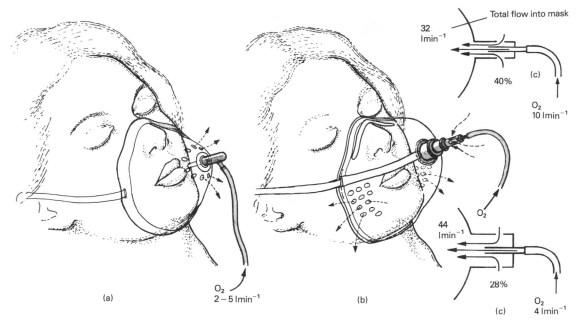

Fig. 12.2 Devices for administration of oxygen. (a) The 'MC' type mask; (b) the air entrainment mask; (c) detail of the air entrainment arrangement for two percentages of oxygen

of inspired oxygen concentration is unnecessary. In the average adult post-operative patient, a flow of 4 l min into the mask results in an FIO_2 of approximately 0.4.

(2) *Air entrainment masks*
If only a small increase in FIO_2 is required but must be precisely known, then an air entrainment or 'constant pressure jet mixing' mask is employed (e.g. Vickers ventimask). Here added oxygen entrains room air through side holes in the mask so that a premixed large flow of oxygen enriched air, of known FIO_2 is presented to the patient. As this usually exceeds maximum inspiratory flow, accurate FIO_2s can be achieved (e.g. 0.24, 0.28 and 0.35, see Fig. 12.2).

Oxygen Toxicity

Although essential to life, prolonged increases in PIO_2 above normal may result in toxicity. This is particularly seen in the premature neonate as retrolental fibroplasia and in the older patient as pulmonary oxygen toxicity.

Pulmonary oxygen toxicity

Oxygen radicals are utilised by the body's defence systems, particularly the polymorphs, for killing harmful microorganisms. This involves the production of free superoxide radicals (O_2 + electron) which are then broken down to hydrogen peroxide by superoxide dismutases, and thence by catalases to oxygen and water. There is evidence that excess oxygen pressures increase superoxide formation and decrease its breakdown by inhibition of superoxide dismutase.

Excess free radicals are normally rendered harmless by scavenging compounds which contain -SH groups. The latter are also affected by high oxygen concentrations which leave the free radicals able to attack cell membrane phospholipids producing lipid peroxidation. This occurs primarily in the lung, presumably as it faces the highest partial pressures. Capillary endothelial damage results, and this leads to interstitial fluid accumulation and reduced compliance with consequent pulmonary failure.

PIO_2 should always be kept below about 40 kPa (300 mmHg, FIO_2 0.4) to reduce the likelihood of this occurring.

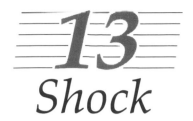

Shock

Definition

Shock is a syndrome characterised by a critical reduction in microcirculatory perfusion. This may be due to a variety of causes, but the end result is cellular dysfunction due to oxygen and nutrient lack. If this process is not reversed before cellular death and multiple organ failure occur, shock becomes irreversible and the patient dies.

Aetiological Classification

There are countless classifications of shock, which try to take account of all the eventualities that may cause the shock syndrome. For simplicity, in this account, shock is divided into three main groups; cardiogenic, hypovolaemic and distributive.

(a) Cardiogenic

Here, it is the primary inability of the heart to pump blood in sufficient quantities to essential capillary beds that results in the reduction in microcirculatory perfusion.

(b) Hypovolaemic

Here, it is a reduction in circulating volume which results in an inadequate cardiac preload. It is the consequent reduction in cardiac output, secondary to peripheral circulatory failure that results in the reduction in microcirculatory perfusion. This may be due to:

1 External fluid loss; this is defined as a loss of blood, plasma or exudate/transudate from the extra- and intracellular compartments, e.g. haematemesis, burn exudate.
2 Internal fluid loss; this is defined as a loss of fluid from the circulating volume into the interstitium, without there necessarily being an overall reduction in extra- and intracellular fluids. This results from an abnormal increase in vascular permeability, e.g. in sepsis and allergy/anaphylaxis.

(c) Distributive

Here circulating volume and cardiac output may be normal or even high, but blood flow bypasses or is redistributed away from essential capillary beds. This 'shunting' results in peripheral circulatory failure and a fall in microcirculatory perfusion. It is classically seen in the early stage of sepsis.

Obviously, in terminal stages of shock, the picture may be mixed.

Clinical Presentation

(a) Categories of patient who present with shock include:

1 Following major trauma and surgery; associated with blood loss, transfusion, bony injury leading to fat embolus, organ dysfunction due to direct injury (e.g. heart, lung and kidney), sepsis, malnutrition, acid-aspiration, and so on.
2 Immunosuppression; associated with leukaemias and lymphomas, cytotoxic drugs, organ transplants, toxic shock, etc.
3 Infection; tuberculosis, malaria, legionella, etc.

4 Miscellaneous; collagen diseases, pre-eclampsia and eclampsia.

The type of shock depends on the primary cause, however, in later stages the reduction in microcirculatory perfusion results in organ failure with similar features despite the differences in aetiology.

(b) Signs of organ dysfunction:
1 Cerebral: confusion, irrational behaviour, altered sensorium leading to progressive coma.
2 Cardiac: hypotension, tachycardia, dysrhythmias, increased core/skin temperature gradient, central and peripheral cyanosis, metabolic acidosis.
3 Pulmonary: tachypnoea, respiratory acidosis and distress, cyanosis.
4 Renal: alteration in osmotic and sodium clearance, usually manifest as oliguria or anuria with progressive azotaemia.
5 Hepatic: jaundice, low albumin, raised enzymes, clotting abnormalities leading to bleeding tendency.
6 Gut: loss of appetite and absorption of enteral feeds, gastrointestinal tract haemorrhage.
7 Skin: pallor, cold and clammy, cyanosis.

Pathophysiology of Shock and Outline of Treatment

(a) Cardiogenic

Primary pump failure may result from myocardial infarction, tamponade, cardiomyopathy, contusion and intractable dysrhythmias. Following infarction or contusion, ischaemic and necrotic muscle is unable to contract adequately and may also be the source of ectopic excitation. Together these lead to a reduction in cardiac efficiency and stroke volume. This also follows failure of ventricular filling in tamponade or primary muscle disease in cardiomyopathy. Thus, despite an adequate ventricular filling pressure, stroke volume is insufficient for adequate microcirculatory perfusion. This also affects the heart itself, so the process rapidly accelerates to the point that cellular acidosis and

organ failure occur. The treatment of cardiac failure and arrest is covered in Chapter 14.

(b) Hypovolaemia due to external fluid loss

Loss of circulating volume produces a variety of compensatory homeostatic responses which are initially protective. A fall in blood pressure stimulates the baroreceptors and leads to increased sympathetic nervous system discharge. Alpha effects increase systemic vascular resistance by reducing blood supply to inessential organ beds, such as skin and splanchnic (but not liver). Sympathetic beta effects increase cardiac contractility and rate, liver and muscle blood flow (major glycogen stores), catecholamine output from the adrenal medulla and renin–angiotensin–aldosterone secretion by effects on the kidney. Reduced atrial pressure, aldosterone and antidiuretic hormone secretion cause a fall in urine output and maximise sodium retention. Reduction in capillary hydrostatic pressure to non-essential capillary beds aids fluid ingress from the interstitial fluid. All these effects maintain microcirculatory perfusion to heart, brain, liver and muscle by diverting circulation to these organs.

Outline of treatment

Immediate, first aid, treatment must ensure that perfusion pressure and oxygen delivery is maintained to vital organs such as brain and heart. Thus, to increase cardiac filling pressure (and thus output and blood pressure) the patient is initially placed head down (bed blocked) and oxygen administered in high concentrations by mask. Exogenous restoration of the appropriate fluid is the mainstay of treatment, e.g. Hartmann's and blood following haemorrhage; 0.9% saline and plasma in burn injury. Adequacy of fluid therapy is guided by clinical signs of restoration of adequate perfusion with reduction of the signs associated with organ dysfunction (see above). In more severe cases it is necessary to measure central venous pressure (CVP) or pulmonary capillary wedge pressure (PCWP) to assess adequacy of fluid replacement and cardiac function. Once patient status has improved, attempts are made to treat the cause of fluid loss.

(c) Hypovolaemia due to internal fluid loss

(1) *Septicaemia* results in release of bacterial endotoxin and abnormal activation of the complement system with massive release of anaphylotoxins (C3a and C5a). This leads to pooling of fluid and a generalised increase in vascular permeability. Initially, this circulatory dilatation is associated with a raised cardiac output (distributive shock), but later the fluid loss leads to a reduction in circulating volume and cold clammy skin and a fall in cardiac output as in internal fluid loss shock. Overactivation of polymorph leucocytes leads to specific endothelial damage especially in the lung. (Endotoxin is a lipopolysaccharide constituent of bacterial cell walls and includes an antigenic fragment known as 'lipid A'. This is held to be responsible for complement activation together with adverse effects on vascular permeability, coagulation and reticuloendothelial function.)

Outline of treatment

In early sepsis, cardiac output is often higher than normal but the tissues are inadequately perfused due to metarteriolar shunting of blood away from essential capillary beds. Treatment is initiated with appropriate antibiotics and the septic focus sought and eradicated. However, the latter may not be obvious, and manipulation and drainage of pus, together with bacterial killing by antibiotics, leads to further endotoxaemia and fluid loss. If treatment is unsuccessful, this stage of 'overwhelming sepsis', characterised by hypotension and warm peripheries, quickly progresses to the later stages of low cardiac output septic shock (vide infra). Administration of large quantities of fluid (0.9% saline and plasma protein fraction, PPF) are necessary together with close monitoring of PCWP and cardiac output. Some of the effects of endotoxaemia, especially that due to bactericidal antibiotics, may be ameliorated by the simultaneous administration of massive doses of corticosteroids (vide infra).

(2) *Allergy/anaphylaxis* again results from release of vasoactive mediators such as histamine, leucotrienes and prostaglandins following exposure of the body's immune system to allergens. The orderly release of these mediators normally aids penetration of leucocytes to eradicate infectious organisms, but in allergy/anaphylaxis there is a widespread uncontrolled release which produces fluid loss, due to increased vascular permeability, and bronchospasm. Four basic types can be identified, anaphylactic (immunoglobulin E-mediated, drugs, allergens), classical and alternate complement activation (e.g. sepsis, endotoxaemia, drugs) and histamine dumping (drugs – usually less severe).

Outline of treatment

The three life-threatening components of allergy/anaphylaxis are: hypotension due to internal fluid loss, oedema which may cause airway obstruction and finally bronchospasm. Any of these may predominate, so initial treatment is directed against the most life-threatening component. Where adequate resuscitation equipment is not close to hand, subcutaneous (or even intravenous) adrenaline is the treatment of choice as this will help maintain cardiac output, reduce bronchospasm and diminish the allergic component. A dose of 1 mg per 70 kg administered subcutaneously (s.c.) or 10 microgram increments i.v. is appropriate. Antihistamines such as chlorpheniramine (10–20 mg s.c., i.m. or i.v. per 70 kg) decrease further fluid loss and oedema. If bronchospasm is the most serious component, aminophylline (250 mg slowly i.v. per 70 kg) and corticosteroids (dexamethasone 4–8 mg i.v. per 70 kg) are appropriate. The latter may also reduce the immune response and particularly airway oedema. If fluid loss is sufficient to cause hypotension (e.g. following thiopentone anaphylaxis) then significant quantities of fluid (1 to 2 litres per 70 kg) have to be administered to restore circulating volume. Both Hartmann's and PPF have been recommended in this situation.

Pathophysiology of Severe Shock

In any of the above situations treatment may be ineffective and this leads to severe or even irreversible shock; e.g. continuing internal fluid loss leads to tissue acidosis and then pooling of blood due to failure of precapillary sphincter tone, initially in non-essential, but eventually in essential organs. Splanchnic ischaemia leads to fluid loss into the bowel and massive release of gut flora endotoxin into the portal venous system. This may overwhelm the 'mopping up' ability of the liver and reticulo-endothelial monocyte macrophage system (REMMS) resulting in systemic endotoxaemia and immunosuppression. The former worsens venous pooling and activates coagulation leading to disseminated intravascular coagulation (DIC), whilst the latter leads to increased risk of sepsis if the patient survives. Apart from the above, liver failure worsens the coagulopathy, and renal failure supervenes at an early stage as a result of the combined effects of vasoconstriction, hypovolaemia and DIC.

REMMS depression as above, and in severe sepsis, allows polymorphs (activated by endotoxaemia directly and via the complement cascade) to attack non-specific essential targets such as pulmonary vascular endothelium, leading to the adult respiratory distress syndrome (ARDS, Chapter 11).

It appears that the 'bridge of irreversibility' is crossed, not only because the body's defence systems are inadequate, but also because the inhibitory mediators that keep these processes in check are consumed. For instance, the coagulation cascade limits blood loss, but also limits, mechanically, lymphatic spread of infection. Consumption of anti-thrombin III, which is inhibitory to most of the activated coagulation factors, leads to uncontrolled coagulation and secondarily, consumptive coagulopathy. Excess products of fibrin degradation, as a result of excessive coagulation, must be inactivated by the macrophage system, which as has been pointed out may be defective in shock from any cause. Fibrin degradation products in excess inhibit clotting and platelet aggregation, and increase vascular permeability further worsening the bleeding tendency (Chapter 6).

Other systems such as the kallikrein and prostaglandin/leucotriene system may be similarly involved.

Therapeutic and Physiological Goals in the Treatment of Shock

Although certain well-defined physiological parameters exist which should be attained in resuscitating 'shocked' patients, e.g. mean blood pressure of about 90 mmHg, central venous pressure of 5–10 cm H_2O, PaO_2 13.3 kPa (100 mmHg), etc., it may be inappropriate rigorously to adhere to a set of values which relate to 'normal' patients during treatment. It is probably more important to accept a mean blood pressure of 60 mmHg, a central venous pressure of 15 and a PaO_2 of only 8 kPa (60 mmHg), provided oxygen delivery and red cell mass are adequate (Chapter 12). As cardiac failure accompanies shock both primarily and secondarily, monitoring PCWP and cardiac output with a flow-directed thermodilution catheter is more appropriate than central venous pressure. It may also avoid the need for inotropes which otherwise might seem necessary where hypotension accompanies a 'normal' central venous pressure but pulmonary wedge pressure is low (Chapter 14). Fluid therapy is more appropriate and restores mean blood pressure and cardiac output.

Massive doses of steroids (e.g. 30 mg kg^{-1} of methylprednisolone 6 hourly for 4 doses) remains controversial but they do have theoretical benefits on improvement of myocardial function, reduction in vascular fluid leak, reduction of anaphylotoxins and leucotrienes, etc. They do not have harmful effects in the short term and should be administered early in the course of shock if they are to be used at all.

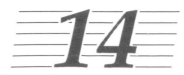

Cardiac failure and cardiac arrest; measurement of filling pressures

Cardiac Failure

Cardiac failure is defined as a primary inability of the heart, as a pump, to provide tissue perfusion which is adequate both to supply nutrients and oxygen to the tissues and to remove waste products. It should be noted that if tissue demands are excessive (e.g. thyrotoxicosis, sepsis) or if blood bypasses tissue beds (e.g. arteriovenous fistulae, Paget's disease of bone and sepsis) then cardiac failure can occur when cardiac output is actually higher than normal (so called 'high output failure').

Pathophysiology

(1) *Anatomical components*
Cardiac failure may arise due to defects in one or more of the anatomical components involved with cardiac contraction and pumping of blood:

Conducting tissue, as in complete heart block, supraventricular dysrhythmias.

Muscle, as in ischaemia, infarction, myopathies, myocarditis, systemic hypertension and electrolyte or blood gas abnormalities.

Arteries, as in thrombosis and arteriosclerosis.

Valves, as in rheumatic heart disease, ruptured chordae and endocarditis.

Chambers, as in atrial and ventricular septal defect and single ventricle.

Pericardium, as in constrictive pericarditis and pericardial effusion.

Disease processes may affect one or more of these components, e.g. infection can affect valves, pericardium and muscle; arteriosclerosis, conducting tissue, muscle and arteries. The mechanisms producing cardiac failure are obviously different, e.g. mitral regurgitation results in volume overload, whilst aortic stenosis and systemic hypertension produce pressure overload, the former being better tolerated in the long term. In addition, chronic changes are better tolerated than acute, e.g. acutely ruptured mitral chordae may produce crushing heart failure, whereas chronic mitral regurgitation may exist with little disability for years.

(2) *Pathophysiology of clinical signs and symptoms*
Cardiac output is the product of stroke volume and heart rate. Stroke volume is determined by three factors:

Preload: this is determined by the venous return to the ventricle and is affected by posture, drugs, volume repletion, muscle venous pump, negative intrathoracic pressure and so on. Increasing the preload increases the end-diastolic fibre length of the ventricular muscle which results in an increased force of contraction (Frank–Starling mechanism).

Afterload: this is the opposition (impedance) to ejection of blood produced by the peripheral circulation (arteries, arterioles and pre-capillary sphincters) to ventricular ejection. For a given contractile state and preload, increasing the afterload (e.g. by arteriolar vasoconstriction) results in a reduced stroke volume.

Contractility: this may be increased by sympathetic nervous system stimulation, exogenous and endogenous catecholamines; and reduced by hypoxia, hypercarbia and acidosis. It means that, for a given pre- and afterload, the stroke volume increases with increasing contractility and vice versa.

Thus, preload and contractility determine the total amount of force of the next cardiac contraction and afterload determines the proportion that must be expended in overcoming impedance and that which can be used to produce useful ejection of blood.

(3) *Compensation*

A reduced cardiac output from any of the mechanisms above means that for a given preload, contractility and afterload, blood flow is insufficient. This leads to compensatory action such as, activation of the sympathetic nervous system, probably via the baroreceptors which increases contractility and heart rate and activates the renin–angiotensin–aldosterone axis. The latter leads to sodium and water retention which increases circulating volume and thereby venous return and preload and is amplified by the decreased renal blood flow as a result of reduced cardiac output. However, a detrimental effect of sympathetic nervous system activation is an increase in afterload. In the short term, there is adequate compensation, but with an inability to increase cardiac output with exercise. In the longer term these effects are deleterious.

Increase in left ventricular preload or end diastolic pressure (LVEDP) causes back pressure to the pulmonary capillaries. This hydrostatic pressure may exceed the plasma oncotic pressure, causing fluid to leak into the lung interstitial space. This reduces pulmonary compliance resulting in dyspnoea, and if severe, causes hypoxia and pulmonary oedema. In addition, in most cases of cardiac failure, blood supply to the myocardium is tenuous, not least from the fact that a low cardiac output reduces its own blood supply directly.

(4) *The importance of oxygen supply/demand*

It is important to maintain (as in the ischaemic myocardium) a positive balance of oxygen supply/demand.

Oxygen demand is determined by:

Wall tension (ventricular pressure/wall thickness × radius, Laplace's law)
Heart rate and contractility

Oxygen supply is determined by:

The product of coronary blood flow and arterial oxygen content

Coronary blood flow (CBF) is equal to coronary perfusion pressure (CPP = diastolic pressure − LVEDP) divided by coronary vascular resistance, and as it occurs predominantly in diastole, is also dependent on diastolic time. The means of determining arterial oxygen content is described in Chapter 12. Thus, it is seen that many of the compensatory mechanisms in cardiac failure produce increases in oxygen demand, e.g. increased rate, contractility, preload (by increasing tension), and some also decrease supply, e.g. increased heart rate decreases time of diastole, and increase in LVEDP decreases CPP. In decompensated cardiac failure, treatment is directed towards the improvement of cardiac output whilst at the same time producing a beneficial increase in the oxygen supply/demand ratio.

Clinical and physiological signs

Cardiac failure may involve the right or left heart, or both. The latter is called congestive cardiac failure (CCF) and the clinical signs and symptoms result from a combination of pulmonary venous congestion (raised LVEDP) and low cardiac output. This produces dyspnoea, i.e. an awareness of the necessity to breathe (a function normally carried out automatically), and must be differentiated from dyspnoea from other causes, such as respiratory disease and anaemia. Classically, there is dyspnoea on exertion and on lying flat (orthopnoea). The latter may become severe enough to awaken the patient (paroxysmal nocturnal dyspnoea). Exertional dyspnoea results not only from a raised LVEDP but also respiratory muscle fatigue due to a combination of increased demand (due to reduced lung compliance) and decreased blood flow (due to low cardiac output). Orthopnoea and paroxysmal nocturnal dyspnoea result from an increase in preload in the recumbent position due to posture together with influx into the circulatory volume of oedema fluid.

On examination, the patient with CCF is dyspnoeic, has cold clammy skin and raised jugular venous pressure (JVP). Predominant right ventricular failure results in increased liver size, ascites and ankle oedema, left ventricular failure (LVF) produces basal crepitations in both lung fields and a third heart sound (gallop rhythm) due to rapid ventricular filling. ECG changes are non-specific but ischaemia and strain pattern is seen with LVF.

Treatment

(1) *The simple case*
In the uncomplicated case of CCF due to mild atheroma and ischaemia, cardiac glycosides (digoxin) may be given to improve contractility and LVEDP is lowered by administration of diuretics which decrease circulating volume. Together with a moderate restriction of activity, this may be sufficient.

(2) *The complicated case*
Acute pulmonary oedema: the patient presents in extremis, hypoxic, dyspnoeic and peripherally shut-down; frothy pink-coloured sputum suggesting that LVEDP is very high. Treatment consists of reassurance firstly, and then reducing the LVEDP. This is achieved by sitting the patient up and administering oxygen, morphine i.v. (venodilator) and frusemide. These simple measures usually suffice if the situation is not too complicated, e.g. as a result of myocardial infarction, rapid dysrhythmias and so on.
Severe or refractory cardiac failure: here it is necessary to resort to invasive monitoring to assess

quantitatively cardiac function. A useful parameter to follow is left ventricular stroke work index (LVSWI).

Work is defined as force times distance moved, and force may be expressed as pressure times area. Thus,

$$Work = pressure \times area \times distance$$

Area times distance has the units of volume. Therefore, work can be calculated as pressure times volume.
It is calculated as follows:

$$LVSWI = (MaBP - PCWP) \times (C.I./heart\ rate) \times 0.0136$$
$$(pressure \times volume)$$

Normally,

$$LVSWI = (90 - 5) \times (4000/80) \times 0.0136$$
$$= 53\ g\ m\ m^{-2}$$
$$(minimum\ in\ the\ adult,\ 20\ g\ m\ m^{-2})$$

MaBP is mean arterial blood pressure, PCWP is pulmonary capillary wedge pressure, C.I. is cardiac index (cardiac output in ml per body surface area in m^2) and multiplying by 0.0136 converts this value into $g\ m\ m^{-2}$. PCWP is measured by a pulmonary artery catheter wedged in a large branch of the pulmonary artery, and it measures back pressure from the left ventricle (approximately LVEDP). The latter is related to left ventricular end diastolic volume (LVEDV) a function of left ventricular preload.

Cardiac output is usually measured by thermodilution techniques but it is a less reliable indicator than LVSWI of cardiac work as it takes no account of heart rate, mean blood pressure or LVEDP (a cardiac output of $5\ l\ min^{-1}$ with a heart rate of 60 is better than one with a rate of 160!).

The required therapy can be determined by reference to the Bolooki box (Fig. 14.1), which relates LVSWI to PCWP. It provides a quick indicator of the position of the patient on the Starling curve which relates cardiac output to filling pressure. PCWP should be kept below 18 mmHg to reduce the possibility of pulmonary oedema.

Thus, in cases where cardiac output is low, values may be obtained in either of the boxes, A, C or D and appropriate treatment results

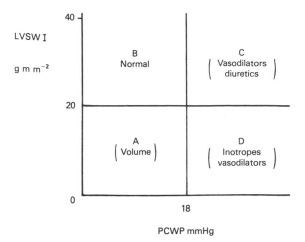

Fig. 14.1 The 'Bolooki Box'. This shows the relationship between pulmonary capillary wedge pressure (PCWP) and left ventricular stroke work index (LVSWI) for therapeutic purposes. Therapeutic manoeuvres appear in brackets

(hopefully) in movement to box B ('normal' with LVSWI > 20 g m m^{-2}, PCWP < 18 mmHg).

> Box A = low LVSWI and low PCWP and requires a cautious fluid challenge to raise LVEDP and preload.
>
> Box C = 'normal' LVSWI and high PCWP. Blood pressure is often normal due to a high systemic vascular resistance (SVR), and this accounts for the 'normal' LVSWI. Appropriate therapy is to reduce PCWP with vasodilators and diuretics.
>
> Box D = the most difficult and complicated case. An improvement in LVSWI by increasing cardiac output is required, together with an overall increase in the MaBP/PCWP ratio. Cardiac output and MaBP are increased by administration of an agent which increases contractility (inotrope), preferably with the major effect on increasing stroke volume and not rate (chronotropy). A suitable agent is dobutamine which is administered as a continuous infusion starting with a rate of about 3 μg kg^{-1} min^{-1}, and increasing as necessary to 20 μg kg^{-1} min^{-1}. However, a concomitant increase in PCWP may occur and this can be reduced with a vasodilator such as sodium nitroprusside.

Cardiac Arrest

Cardiac arrest is defined as a reduction in cardiac output which is so severe that blood flow to vital organs is critically compromised. Unless an effective cardiac output can be restored immediately, death will supervene in a matter of minutes. It results from dysrhythmias such as ventricular tachycardia or fibrillation (VT or VF), very rapid supraventricular dysrhythmias, complete heart block or asystole. These often occur at the end stage of serious cardiac dysfunction, e.g. severe infarct, massive haemorrhage and sepsis. Thus, treatment also includes the underlying condition, e.g. volume replacement, correction of electrolyte or blood gas disturbances.

Outline of treatment

When faced with a patient suffering from cardiac arrest from any cause, it is important to have a well-defined plan and execute it expeditiously. A commonly used protocol is the A, B and C. Thus:

A = Airway. Vomitus and false teeth must be removed and the airway made patent.

B = Breathing. Ascertain if the patient is breathing, as often the patient is suffering from a respiratory arrest (e.g. post-operative) and simple mechanical ventilation is all that is required. In true cardiac arrest, breathing will have stopped and the patient must be ventilated, either mouth-to-mouth, via a Brook airway, or preferably with 100% oxygen via a reservoir bag (Ambu or Waters) and face mask.

C = Circulation. Check the carotid and femoral pulses and apex beat, they may be present as in B. If not, start external cardiac massage (ECM) by putting the patient on a firm surface and placing one hand on the lower end of the sternum and the other on top and aiming to compress the sternum about 2–3 cm 70 times per minute. In babies the chest is compressed with the thumb. It may be worth giving one fist thump over the sternum at this stage as occasionally VF (the most common cause) will revert to sinus rhythm.

If one is single handed, give one breath of oxygen or expired air for every 10 compressions. Once assistance has arrived, the patient is intubated (to aid ventilation and prevent aspiration of gastric contents), ECM is continued, an intravenous infusion is established and the ECG monitored. It is now accepted that sodium bicarbonate in all but the smallest amounts is detrimental, so only about 25–50 mmol may be given, hyperventilating the patient to reduce respiratory acidosis, and blood pH checked. As this is occurring the ECG is observed. VF is treated with a DC shock of 300 joules (less in children) with the paddles over the sternum and apex and repeated if ineffective. If the VF is very fine, coarsen it with 0.1 ml kg^{-1} of 1:10,000 adrenaline i.v., not intracardiac. Often sinus rhythm occurs but the patient reverts to VF or VT in which case lignocaine 1 mg kg^{-1} followed by an infusion of 2–4 mg kg^{-1} h^{-1} is often effective. In cases of resistant VF, bretyllium 5–10 mg kg^{-1} may be given i.v. as a last resort. If the rhythm reverts to sinus bradycardia, atropine 20 μg kg^{-1} is administered i.v. (1.2 mg in the 60 kg adult). Complete heart block is initially treated with isoprenaline followed by pacing, which can now satisfactorily be applied externally or via the oesophagus.

Asystole is less common, and must be converted into VF with adrenaline. Supraventricular dysrhythmias are treated with DC shock but the output should not exceed 50 joules. During this time ECM and IPPV is continued, although it should be realised that cardiac output in these circumstances is less than $\frac{1}{3}$ normal, so perfusion to vital organs, particularly the brain, is markedly reduced. Pupil signs should not be used as a determinant of discontinuing support as they are distinctly unreliable, rather it is determined by the medical team present and the patient's history.

It should be noted that modern defibrillator equipment has the provision for ECG monitoring via the paddles when placed in position for defibrillation. This considerably speeds up diagnosis of the dysrhythmia.

Other drugs commonly used are calcium chloride (5 mmol boluses) and isoprenaline (apart from complete heart block). No convincing evidence has accumulated to favour the former, indeed calcium antagonists may be beneficial in reducing myocardial and cerebral damage following arrest.

Measurement of Cardiac Filling Pressures

(a) Central Venous Pressures (CVP)

In the shocked, traumatised or anaesthetised patient, maintenance of normal cardiac output and organ blood flow is an essential prerequisite to a satisfactory clinical outcome (Chapter 13). Measurement of cardiac output is not always possible in the clinical setting, so arterial blood pressure is often used as a guideline. If arterial blood pressure should fall during major surgery, for example, it may be difficult to decide whether this fall is due to a reduction in cardiac output as a result of cardiac depression or an inadequate filling pressure. In most patients who do not have intrinsic heart disease, measurement of central venous pressure (CVP) enables the clinician to distinguish between the former, where CVP will be normal or high, and the latter where it will be low. However, in difficult or equivocal cases, pulmonary capillary wedge pressures (PCWP) obtained from a flow directed pulmonary artery catheter provides more accurate information (vide infra).

Measurements of CVP are usually taken in cm of water (occasionally in mm of mercury); SI units are not in clinical use at present.

Technique
CVP refers to the pressure of venous blood in the superior vena cava or right atrium, i.e. the filling pressure or preload of the right ventricle. To measure this pressure it is necessary to place a catheter or cannula so that its tip lies, usually, in the superior vena cava. This catheter is filled with saline or dextrose, so as to form a continuous fluid 'bridge' with the measuring device (Fig. 14.2). Placement of the CVP line in the superior vena cava demands considerable expertise, and may be carried out in the following ways:

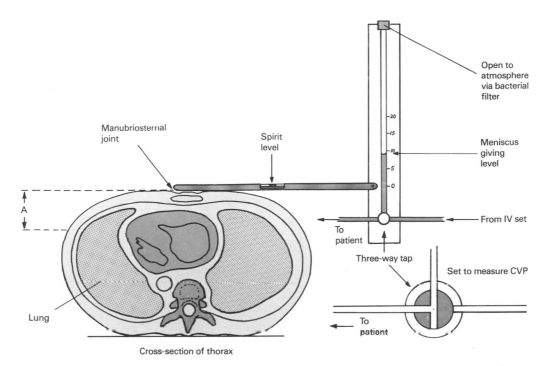

Manubriosternal joint

Spirit level

Open to atmosphere via bacterial filter

Meniscus giving level

-20
-15
-10
-5
-0

From IV set

To patient

Three-way tap

Set to measure CVP

To patient

A

Lung

Cross-section of thorax

Fig. 14.2 Arrangement of CVP measuring system. As shown, CVP zero is conventionally taken from the manubrio-sternal joint, whereas the 'actual' level is lower. This difference, which is shown as 'A' on the diagram, is about 5–10 cmH$_2$O. Thus, in some normal subjects, CVP may have a negative value (see text). The insert shows the position of the 3-way tap whilst the CVP is being measured

(1) *Via the median cubital vein at the elbow:*
This is the route that should be used by inexperienced clinicians, as it is associated with the least morbidity. A suitable 60 cm catheter (in the adult) is selected and is advanced through a previously inserted cannula under sterile conditions. Advancing the catheter may be difficult due to obstructions in the vein, particularly at the shoulder region. It may be necessary to get an assistant to bring the arm out to a right angle whilst the catheter is manipulated through to the central veins. Alternative methods include turning the head from side to side, injecting saline whilst advancing the catheter, and so on. In some cases it may be impossible to reach the superior vena cava by this route. Correct positioning of the catheter is determined clinically by estimating the length inserted and confirmed by X-ray.
(2) *Via the external jugular vein:*
The patient is tipped head down and the head is then turned to the left. A pillow may be

inserted under the shoulder. The right external jugular vein is chosen as this presents the straightest passage into the superior vena cava. A shorter catheter/cannula combination, e.g. 30 cm is chosen. The saline filled catheter is advanced through the cannula that was previously inserted into the external jugular vein. Considerable difficulty may be experienced in persuading the catheter to pass through the pair of valves and the oblique angle between the external jugular vein and the subclavian vein into which it drains. A 'J' tipped guide wire is often necessary for this manoeuvre. Again, the catheter tip placement should be confirmed by X-ray.
(3) *Via the internal jugular vein and subclavian vein:*
For consistent and reliable superior vena cava catheterisation the internal jugular and subclavian veins on the right side are used. However, their deep location means that vital structures may be punctured during attempts at

cannulation, e.g. carotid and subclavian arteries, pleura and so on. The complication rate is sufficiently high and serious enough to preclude this route in all but the most experienced hands. Technical aspects are beyond the scope of this book.

Obtaining the CVP reading
Once catheter tip placement has been confirmed, a saline manometer is connected to its luer connection. This is arranged as in Fig. 14.2. Zero is taken to be at the level of the manubriosternal joint with the patient lying horizontally, a spirit level often being used for accurate alignment. The vertical limb of the manometer is filled to the top from the bag by appropriately turning the three way tap. The latter is then turned in the direction of the catheter, so that the level in the vertical limb will fall rapidly until it equilibrates with CVP. On reaching this level there should be significant respiratory fluctuation of the meniscus level. This confirms that the catheter is in free communication with the superior vena cava. Failure to do so means that the reading will be inaccurate. The catheter is continuously flushed with fluid to maintain patency, except during CVP measurement.

The normal CVP
The manubriosternal joint is often used as a surface marker for the level of the right atrium because it is the simplest anatomical reference site. In the supine position it is above atrial level by between 5 and 10 cm, and thus values obtained may be negative in the normal patient (Fig. 14.2). It is reasonable to transfuse fluid to a value of +2 to +5 cmH$_2$O in the hypovolaemic patient. A value of more than +5 indicates that the patient is not fluid depleted, and if associated with hypotension, suggests that an element of this is due to cardiac depression.

Clinical use of the CVP
The CVP gives important information about the patient's blood volume, particularly with regard to fluid therapy. Fluid depletion may not be reflected in a low blood pressure if the patient is awake, anxious and tachycardic, e.g. in perforated duodenal ulcer. However, ablation of

sympathetic drive with increased peripheral vascular resistance, which is helping to maintain arterial blood pressure, by administration of general anaesthesia may result in cardiovascular collapse. Insertion of a CVP catheter would have revealed a low reading and allowed adequate fluid replacement to take place prior to surgery.

(b) Pulmonary capillary wedge pressure (PCWP)

Blood pressure and cardiac output are mainly functions of the ability of the left ventricle (LV) to pump blood. In a healthy patient subjected to moderate fluid and blood loss, fluid status can be fairly accurately obtained by clinical signs of adequate perfusion, blood pressure and measurement of CVP which represents the filling pressure and function of the right ventricle. This usually correlates accurately with the LV filling pressures, but in very sick patients, especially those with poor LV function, this close correlation is lost. Attempting to increase CVP in such patients only results in excessive blood being pumped into the LV with raised PCWP and pulmonary oedema. Thus, if raising the CVP does not produce a satisfactory increase in blood pressure and clinical status, PCWP (a close correlate of LV filling pressures) must be measured.

The pioneering work of Swan and Ganz has enabled catheters to be placed into the pulmonary artery (PA). This is possible by the provision of a balloon placed at its tip which can be inflated when the catheter enters the right ventricle. This helps to carry the catheter into the PA where it wedges in one of its larger branches. Once the catheter is wedged, it no longer measures the pressure in the pulmonary artery, but the back pressure from the left atrium and pulmonary capillaries. This may be used to determine LV function as indicated above.

(c) Conclusion

Hypovolaemia is frequently underestimated in the patient presenting for emergency surgery. If inadequately treated it is often only recognised when the patient suffers profound cardiovascular collapse at induction of anaesthesia.

Clinical estimates of adequacy of circulating volume such as skin perfusion, moistness of tongue and urine output usually provide sufficient information so that hypovolaemia can be appropriately treated. In severe depletion, or when there is continuing rapid fluid loss, measurement of CVP is the only safe guide to infusion therapy. In cases of suspected LV failure as an additional cause of hypotension, despite an adequate CVP, a pulmonary artery catheter must be inserted to assess LV function.

15

Intensive care problems

The Intensive Care Unit

The Intensive Care Unit is normally referred to as the ICU. It is a special ward with a 1:1 (or higher) nurse to patient ratio, and, in most units, a registrar grade anaesthetist available round the clock. Each bed has (or should have) a set of monitoring and supporting equipment for the circulatory, respiratory and renal systems. Hospitals serving large population groups have, in addition to a general ICU, other more specialised wards. They provide care for premature and sick new-born babies (Special Care Baby Unit – SCBU), post-myocardial infarction patients (Coronary Care Unit – CCU), neurosurgical or renal failure patients. In most general ICUs average patient stay is of the order of 4–6 days, with a large contribution from postoperative surgical patients. The number of beds may be as low as 2 or as high as 24, but most have 6 to 8 beds. The nurses are specially trained, and there is additional technical staff to provide on site maintenance and calibration of monitoring and life-support equipment.

The simplest set of equipment for each bed consists of the following:

Electrocardiogram (ECG) monitor with printout
Pressure monitors for measurement and display of arterial and venous pressures, together with a conventional sphygmomanometer
Skin and core temperature monitor
Ventilator
Compressed air and oxygen; suction
Blood warmer
Intravenous infusion controller

In addition, the ward should have the following equipment on site:

Blood-gas analyser
K^+/Na^+ analyser
Osmometer
One or more cardiac arrest trolleys with defibrillators
Tracheal intubation trolley with anaesthetic drugs sufficient for induction of anaesthesia.

This chapter will outline the management of a few situations often seen in ICUs.

Trauma

Patients surviving severe trauma are usually admitted to ICU. Injuries producing massive blood loss are not discussed here; blood replacement is dealt with in Chapter 6.

The situations more commonly seen are:

(a) Multiple trauma

Patients in this category are those with injuries inflicted on more than one system. A common combination is multiple bone fractures associated with a head injury and/or crush injury of the chest. Multiple bone fractures may be the cause of 'fat embolism syndrome', of which adult respiratory distress syndrome (ARDS) is a component (Chapter 11). This consists of acute respiratory failure, with predominantly an hypoxic component (initially $PaCO_2$ may be low) often associated with neurological symptoms such as disorientation followed by stupor and occasionally coma. It is thought to be due to a complex chain of events initiated by complement activation triggered within the injured tissue or by factors released into the circulation.

(b) Head injuries

Patients with head injuries admitted to ICU are usually unconscious. The main points in the management are:

Firstly, frequent assessment and adequate monitoring of the neurological state and cardiorespiratory systems

Secondly, adoption of measures to prevent intracranial pressure (ICP) from rising, or to lower it if already high.

Cardiorespiratory monitoring and neurological assessment are mandatory because they provide the only clues as to the worsening of the condition, which may happen very rapidly. Any respiratory or circulatory complication arising after admission will make the neurological situation worse. Permanent neurological damage may result from the initial injury, but it is often due to events occurring post trauma. The main component appears to be increased ICP as a result of haematoma (which needs urgent surgical evacuation) or acute oedema of the brain. The latter is a non-specific tissue response to injury leading to increased ICP which may be severe enough to cause permanent ischaemic damage. Thus, continuous routine intracranial pressure monitoring, through a burr hole, is the best guide for therapy aimed at lowering it.

The most important factors determining ICP are $PaCO_2$, arterial pressure and temperature. Management includes general supportive measures such as maintenance of fluid, electrolyte and caloric balance, bladder catheterisation and maintenance of the airway.

Specific measures to decrease intracranial pressure include:

1 Administration of mannitol $1\,g\,kg^{-1}$ i.v. on admission, and (debatably) up to a further three similar doses at 12 hour intervals.
2 The patient should be mechanically ventilated at a minute volume sufficient to drop $PaCO_2$ to approximately 3.7 kPa (28 mmHg). A neuromuscular blocker is administered regularly to prevent reflex contraction of res-

piratory muscles leading to peaks of very high intrathoracic pressure. These are partly transmitted to the brain through the internal jugular veins. PaO_2 should be 150 mmHg (20 kPa).
3 Prevention and treatment of any rise of core temperature above 37°C.
4 Prevention and treatment of any rise in mean arterial blood pressure above 100 mmHg.
5 Sedation with anxiolytic/anaesthetic agents to reduce cerebral metabolic rate especially if cerebral perfusion is compromised.

Glasgow Coma Scale

This is the prototype assessment of neurological status and is based on a 15 point scale:

EYE OPENING	Score
Spontaneous	4
To speech	3
To pain	2
None	1

BEST MOTOR RESPONSE	
Obeys	6
Localises	5
Withdraws	4
Abnormal flexion	3
Extensor	2
None	1

BEST VERBAL RESPONSE	
Orientated	5
Confused	4
Inappropriate words	3
Incomprehensible	2
None	1

TOTAL (maximum)	15

90% of head injured patients with a score greater than 11 on admission recover some useful neurological function in time (6 months to a year). Of those with a score less than 4, 90% remain severely brain damaged (vegetative).

(c) Chest injuries

Crush injuries of the chest are common; if there is rupture of the great vessels they are often fatal. Haemo and/or pneumothorax, broncho-pleural fistula and rupture of the diaphragm usually require pleural drainage and/or surgical treatment; haemopericardium is a surgical emergency.

Rib fractures with contusion of the lung or with a flail segment usually lead to severe respiratory failure demanding mechanical ventilation (IPPV). This should be applied for a minimum of two weeks to allow the ribs to stabilise. If the endotracheal tube has been inserted through the nose, it is possible to maintain these patients on the ventilator without administration of muscle relaxants and with a minimum of sedation.

(d) Acute renal failure

A frequent accompaniment of trauma and sepsis in the ICU patient is acute renal failure (ARF). It is a complication best avoided as it carries a high morbidity and mortality, especially if combined with failure of other organs. The causes are multifactorial and include:

1 Blood loss with severe hypovolaemia and hypotension. Here the body responds to a loss of circulating volume by maximal sodium and water retention (Chapter 13). Although blood pressure may be normal, this is at the expense of profound vasoconstriction associated with a reduced cardiac output and renal blood flow. The urine output is low (<0.5 ml kg^{-1} h^{-1}) and has the characteristics of pre-renal oliguria, i.e. Na less than 20 mmol l^{-1} and an osmolality of at least twice that of serum. The central venous pressure (CVP) should be measured and fluid repletion continued until it is at least 5 cm H$_2$O. If this does not produce an increase in urine output, 0.5 g kg^{-1} of mannitol are given followed by dopamine 2–3 μg kg^{-1} min^{-1} (a dose which specifically increases renal blood flow). Loop diuretics such as frusemide should not be administered unless it is unequivocally established that the patient is fluid repleted. Administration of frusemide to the fluid-depleted patient may produce what seems to be a satisfactory diuresis, but it worsens the underlying condition and may actually precipitate ARF.
2 Sepsis is often associated with oliguria for a variety of reasons. In the early stages (Chapter 13) there is hypotension with increased cardiac output and dilated peripheries. Renal blood flow is probably abnormally distributed leading to adequate quantity but not quality of urine. The Na content is 20–40 mmol l^{-1} (normal > 60) and the osmolality about 1:1 with plasma. During later stages of septic shock, the cardiac output falls thus lowering renal blood flow. In addition, disseminated intravascular coagulation may cause microthrombosis and renal shut down. It is often necessary in such patients to administer 'best guess' antibiotic therapy as the condition cannot wait for the results of blood culture. This therapy often includes the aminoglycosides, and they are often administered without due regard to their reduced clearance in the already renally compromised patient. The toxic levels achieved often represent the final straw for the kidney and ARF supervenes, especially if aminoglycosides are combined with frusemide.

Treatment and management

This hinges on prevention by consideration of the factors in (1) and (2). Adequate repletion of fluid and blood with measurement of CVP, treatment of sepsis with non-toxic antibiotics (such as cephalosporins), correction of acidosis and normalising serum albumin are the main stays of therapy.

Other Situations Requiring Mechanical Ventilation

Several neurological or neuromuscular syndromes cause respiratory muscle paralysis necessitating ventilatory support. Poliomyelitis has already been mentioned in the historical notes as having contributed to the stimulus leading to development and manufacture of ventilators. Other forms of polyneuritis, such as the Guillain–Barré syndrome, cause similar respiratory problems requiring temporary ventilatory support.

Myasthenia gravis is a disease that interests most anaesthetists because of its similarity to pharmacological neuromuscular blockade.

Indeed the diagnosis and chronic treatment uses the same tools as the management of therapeutic neuromuscular blockade.

Other diseases such as tetanus and status epilepticus can only be managed if neuromuscular transmission is blocked, and mechanical ventilation applied.

All the situations just referred to may be accompanied by severe dysfunction of the autonomic nervous system, leading to dysrhythmias and variations in vasomotor tone.

With the exception of epilepsy, all the other situations share a common problem, that is, the preservation of consciousness of the patient while treatment proceeds. It is not in the best interest of the patient to administer sufficient sedative or anaesthetic drugs to maintain total unconsciousness for periods as long as 10 or 12 weeks, because of the unforeseen effects of such therapy. Instead, everything should be done to provide physical comfort and the development of ways of understanding the patient's requests when only a small group of muscles are functioning. Much is learnt from the experiences of patients that have recovered totally after an episode of total paralysis; regular and frequent turning on the bed, quiet environment, daily news about the patient's improving condition, frequent home news, radio, recorded music or stories are all very important factors in mitigating the patient's suffering.

Failure of Temperature Regulation

Extreme cases of hyperthermia or accidental hypothermia are usually managed in the ICU.

Normal human core temperature is 37°C, and for practical purposes it can be taken as the temperature of arterial blood leaving the aorta. In man this is very close to the temperature of the hypothalamus, where the main temperature regulation centres are sited. Temperature measured in the ear canal, adjacent to the tympanic membrane, is the closest to that of the hypothalamus. Core temperatures above 42°C are fatal due to coagulation of intracellular proteins. Below 30°C there is a high chance of ventricular fibrillation.

Thermoregulatory reflexes arise from the hypothalamus, which contains two groups of neurons, anterior and posterior. The anterior group is concerned with heat loss control and the posterior with heat generation and conservation. Certain substances have been shown to act in these regions, such as noradrenaline, 5-hydroxytryptamine and prostaglandins E_1 and E_2. There are other structures within the central nervous system (spinal cord and brain stem) which contribute to the thermoregulatory reflexes. The only specific thermal receptors known (warm and cold) are in the skin, spinal cord, and hypothalamus.

There is a concept of 'set point' which is the value of core temperature at which the thermoregulatory reflexes are least active. In disease, this control point may be moved up by microbial toxins or other factors causing fever. Some antipyrexial agents (e.g. aspirin, paracetamol) seem to act by inhibiting local prostaglandin activity.

Mechanisms of temperature control

(1) *Heat gain*
Basal metabolism produces heat constantly, and voluntary muscle activity releases more heat as a by-product. Specific heat gaining/conserving mechanisms include behavioural responses (seeking warmer environment, clothing, posture), vasoconstriction of the skin, shivering and increased release of thyroid and medullary adrenal hormones. In the new born the breakdown of brown fat, mediated by noradrenaline, contributes significantly to heat production.

(2) *Heat loss*
Heat is lost through the skin by radiation, convection, conduction and evaporation. In the adult, evaporation is by far the most effective in eliminating excess heat. A small amount of heat is lost with excretions and by evaporation through the lung. Heat loss mechanisms include behavioural responses (such as removing layers of clothing), skin vasodilatation and sweating.

Temperature disturbances

It is evident from the last few paragraphs that patients under anaesthesia, heavily sedated or under neuromuscular blockade cannot control their temperature properly. The important behavioural responses are abolished, and most sedative drugs and anaesthetics attenuate the hypothalamic mechanisms.

(1) *Hyperthermia*
This is usually caused by infection. In the anaesthesia/ICU context it may be caused by accidental overheating due to breakdown of control of heating blankets, by the use of atropine in hot climates or childhood pyrexias (sweating is abolished), or as a result of a rare complication of anaesthesia called 'malignant hyperthermia'. The latter is a form of myopathy that usually remains asymptomatic until an anaesthetic is given. It is related to a defect in the restoration of the calcium balance after muscle contraction. Many of the anaesthetic drugs can trigger the syndrome; suxamethonium and halothane top the list. It is treated with active cooling, IPPV and oxygen, and dantrolene (a drug that restores the calcium balance).

(2) *Hypothermia*
This is nearly always accidental (it may, however, be the presenting feature in myxoedema). It may result from exposure; old people are more susceptible because the heat generating mechanisms are less effective; children are also more susceptible because of the high surface area to weight ratio of the body.

Treatment is conservative, and it is best to allow natural mechanisms to warm up the body slowly. Plasma electrolytes and acid–base balance should be monitored during rewarming as serious disturbances are occasionally seen.

Parenteral and Enteral Feeding

Chapter 6 dealt with intravenous fluid requirements in the peri-operative period. Although regimes containing basically electrolytes with few (but crucial) calories are reasonable for the average patient, after a few days it is essential that the 'normal' nutritional intake is resumed. This problem is magnified in ITU where patients are unable to feed normally for a variety of

reasons, such as unconsciousness, presence of endotracheal tube, gut pathology, etc. Failure to provide adequate nutrition leads to protein catabolism, weight loss, lowered resistance to infection, and eventually death due to inanition.

Normal requirements

These are basically divided into: water, electrolytes, calories, nitrogen, lipid- and water-soluble vitamins and trace elements.

(1) *Water and electrolytes*
These were covered in Chapter 6.

(2) *Energy (calories or kjoules)*
These are provided as glucose and lipids (in a ratio of about 6:4), $130-170 \text{ kJ kg}^{-1}$ or $30-40 \text{ kcal kg}^{-1}$).

(3) *Nitrogen*
1 g of nitrogen is equivalent to 6 g of protein. The minimum requirement is 0.15 g kg^{-1} of N_2 (1 g kg^{-1} of protein).

(4) *Lipid and water-soluble vitamins and trace elements*
Suitable commercial preparations are available which provide adequate quantities of these substances (e.g. Solivito, Vitilipid and Addamel R). It is particularly important to ensure that intake of B_{12}, folic acid, iron, calcium, phosphate, magnesium and zinc are maintained during prolonged periods of parenteral nutrition.

A suitable regime

As water and calorie requirements are roughly similar ($30-40 \text{ ml/kcal kg}^{-1}$ in the adult), the solutions should contain about 4 kJ (1 cal) ml^{-1}. Glucose solutions must therefore exceed 25% (25 g or 4 kJ (1 cal) ml^{-1}), and as this is 5 times the normal serum tonicity, infusion via a large central vein is necessary to avoid thrombophlebitis. Fat (e.g. Intralipid 10% R, 10 g or 380 kJ 100 ml^{-1}) is much less traumatic to veins, but is usually infused through the same site. Nitrogen is administered as an amino acid solution containing the average adult requirement (9 g) in about 1 litre of solution.

TABLE 15.1. Example of parenteral feeding regime

Bottle no. (500 ml)	Product name	kJ	kcal	N$_2$ g	Na$^+$ mmol	K$^+$	Vitamins and trace elements
1	Vamin glucose	1250	300	5	25	10	
2	Dextrose 20%	1700	400				Solivito 10 ml
3	Vamin glucose	1250	300	5	25	10	
4	Intralipid 10%	2100	500				Vitilipid 10 ml
5	Dextrose 20%	1700	400				Addamel 10 ml
Total	2500		8000	1900	10	50	20

A starter regime for a 60 kg man (e.g. third post-operative day) is shown in Table 15.1

Additional Na$^+$ and K$^+$ are administered as necessary. Bottles 1 and 2, and 3 and 4 should run concurrently. Hourly estimations of blood glucose reveal the necessity for insulin (especially septic patients). Prior to administration of lipid, blood should be spun down and observed to be clear (no lipaemia) following the previous infusion. The maximum amount of fat administered should be about 3 g kg^{-1} day (i.e. about 110 kJ (25 kcal) kg^{-1}) and dextrose 7 g kg^{-1} day^{-1} (i.e. about 110 kJ (25 kcal) kg^{-1}).

Setting up

A special central line is necessary for intravenous feeding, inserted under aseptic conditions. This is usually inserted via the subclavian vein into the superior vena cava. In many hospitals, the daily requirements are prescribed and the infusion prepared daily under aseptic conditions by the pharmacist as a single '3 litre bag'. This makes the infusion easier and is said to reduce infection.

Enteral feeding

In most cases, parenteral feeding is unnecessary, as although the patient may be unable to swallow, the gut is working. Many commercial preparations are available, most containing about 4 kJ (1 kcal) ml^{-1} with all the necessary vitamins and trace elements. To ensure absorption in the initial stages they should be administered in small quantities with frequent test aspiration via a large nasogastric tube. However, once absorption is established, a small bore (East Grinstead) tube is inserted into the stomach. This is better tolerated by the patient and causes less trauma to the oesophagus. Placement should be verified by X-ray prior to feeding and its position checked on a daily basis.

16
Management of burns and poisoning

Burns

The spectrum of burn injury is obviously great, ranging from a minor scald to the whole body surface. Treatment of major burn injury, accompanied as it often is by renal and pulmonary failure, represents one of the greatest challenges to intensive care, surgical, nursing and rehabilitatory management.

Pathophysiology

(1) Skin
This is the largest organ in the body and is mainly responsible for water and temperature regulation. It forms an effective barrier to infective organisms. Loss of skin integrity on a large enough scale leads to water loss, failure of temperature regulation, infection of the burn eschar and subsequent sepsis. The area of skin directly affected is coagulated with surrounding viable hyperaemic skin and beyond that erythema. If all dermal elements are destroyed the burn is described as 'full thickness', is insensible to pinprick and requires split skin grafting at a later stage. If some or all of the dermal elements remain, the burn is described as partial thickness (superficial or deep) and heals without the necessity for split skin grafting although this may be necessary for cosmetic or functional reasons.

(2) Respiratory system
Burns of the head and neck frequently give rise to upper airway obstruction due to oedema. This may be sudden, so equipment and expertise for endotracheal intubation or tracheostomy must be to hand. Following smoke or noxious fumes inhalation, the lower respiratory tract and alveoli may be affected leading to adult respiratory distress syndrome (Chapter 11).

(3) Fluid loss
The burn injury results in the release of a number of vasoactive compounds which cause vasodilation and increased vascular permeability (e.g. histamine, bradykinin and prostaglandins). This leads to fluid loss at the site of injury which is obvious, but also fluid loss (oedema) internally, which is not. This, together with red cell destruction can quickly produce hypovolaemia, external fluid loss 'shock' (Chapter 13). Thus, intravenous fluids are extremely important in resuscitation.

(4) Metabolic
Following burn injury, there is a marked increase in metabolic rate and this persists for many days or even weeks. The result is an increased requirement for enteral feeds and also drugs. A reduction can be achieved by nursing the patient in a warm (32°) environment.

(5) Depressed immune response
Following major burn injury, the patient's immune response is depressed. This leads to a high incidence of infection which demands scrupulous asepsis when in contact with this group of patients. It can be several months before the immune response is restored to normality.

Assessment of the burned patient

In the UK, most severe burns (more than 20% of body surface area) are eventually referred to a specialist burns centre, who also advise on appropriate treatment. In this discussion, therefore, only the initial management is dealt with.

(1) *History*

Past medical history should be sought, e.g. cardiorespiratory conditions which could prejudice survival, epilepsy and diabetic hypoglycaemia which could have resulted in the injury. A patient who is recovered unconscious from a smoke-filled room is a likely candidate for an inhalation injury. The time of the burn must be obtained as accurately as possible, as this influences fluid management.

(2) *Examination*

Firstly assess the patient for associated injuries and then obtain the weight. Head and neck burns, charred hair and nasal vibrissae, together with a positive history all suggest the possibility of airway problems. At an early stage, cardiovascular and neurological status will be fairly normal, even after a major burn. This may lead to a false sense of security as the situation is rapidly deteriorating by the minute. One of the most difficult tasks is estimating the size of the burn, as this influences fluid management and the potential for survival.

The 'rule of nines' is most useful (Fig. 16.1). The body is divided into 11 areas of 9%, e.g. the head (1 × 9), arms (2 × 9), back (2 × 9) and front (2 × 9) of the trunk, legs (2 × 2 × 9) and the perineum 1%. Do not count erythema; patchy areas may be calculated by considering that the area of the patient's outstretched hand is equal to 1%. In the child, the head is relatively bigger and the legs smaller. Add all the percentages up to get the total body surface area burned. Note full and partial thickness loss, if possible.

(3) *Investigations*

Take blood for haemoglobin, urea and electrolytes, cross matching, carbon monoxide levels and osmolality. Urine osmolality is also measured. Swab all burned areas for micro-

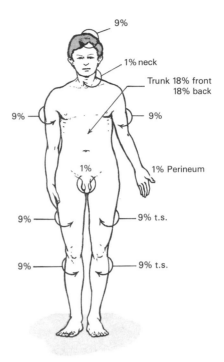

Fig. 16.1 Rule of 'nines' to estimate body surface area burnt, as a percentage of total body surface

organism identification to cover possibility of burn infection.

Treatment of the burn patient

(1) *Airway*

This has been mentioned previously. Be vigilant!

(2) *Intravenous fluids*

Fluid loss due to local exudate and generalised oedema is massive in major burns. It starts from the moment of injury and is proportional to the percentage body surface area (BSA) burned and the weight of the patient. If this exceeds 20% the fluid must be given intravenously. A reliable intravenous access is of paramount importance, make sure it is adequate and firmly strapped in.

The formula usually applied in the UK is Muir and Barclay's, i.e.

% BSA burned × weight in kg/2

to give the 'Unit volume' in ml. This is transfused as plasma protein fraction (PPF) or, cheaper, PPF and gelatin, in 6 periods of 4, 4, 4, 6, 6 and 12 hours respectively. For example, a 60 kg man with 40% burn will have a unit volume of 1200 ml, so he will get 7200 ml (6 × 1200) of PPF and gelatin in 36 hours. In addition, free water as dextrose saline (Na 30 mmol l^{-1}) is also administered for normal metabolic requirements at a rate of 1500 ml m^{-2} 24 h^{-1}.

(3) *Monitoring*
At all times the adequacy of the amount of fluid in (2) is checked by frequent assessment of haematocrit (Hct), urine output and osmolality, overall skin perfusion, blood pressure, mental orientation and so on. A rising Hct suggests inadequate fluids as does a urine output of less than 1 ml kg^{-1} h^{-1} with a high osmolality. Muscle injury following electrical burns frequently results in acute renal failure which may require haemodialysis.

(4) *Analgesia and sedation*
Despite the obvious distress and extent of injury, analgesia and sedation are not urgently required. However, small intravenous increments of morphine are very useful especially when burned clothes are being removed, intravenous infusion is being organised, and dressings are being applied. I.m. injection is unreliable.

(5) *Clean and dress*
As most major burns will be transferred, it is only necessary to clean off obvious contaminants with cetrimide and chlorhexidine (Savlon R). Prophylactic antibiotics are no longer universally administered, but tetanus prophylaxis should be given.

(6) *Escharotomy*
Circumferential burns of the legs, arms, chest wall and neck may cause venous obstruction as oedema fluid accumulates. In severe cases this can result in gangrene in the former two or respiratory obstruction in the latter. A longitudinal incision is made at right angles to the circumferential obstruction so that the tension may be relieved. This manoeuvre may be accompanied by severe haemorrhage.

(7) *Transfer*
Following resuscitation the patient is transferred by ambulance to the burns centre. This may be a journey of a few hours so skilled medical help must be provided for the journey and active fluid resuscitation continued. The patient should be kept warm, given additional oxygen and intravenous analgesics, and facilities must be available for intubation/tracheostomy.

Late management

Following reception at the burns centre, much of the above will be repeated, and the patient transferred to a heated room. The surgical team assesses the need for early operation to remove the burn eschar by tangential excision to reduce the risk of infection, and to take split skin grafts from unburned areas for cover. High volume enteral feeding will be necessary to cover metabolic requirements. Periods of sepsis are treated with appropriate systemic antibiotics, and the patient gradually rehabilitated as the burn heals. Overall, the patient will remain in hospital for about 1 month for every 10% BSA burn, and in major burn injury will require many more admissions for cosmetic and functional plastic surgery in the years to come.

Acute Poisoning

Cases of poisoning account for 1% of hospital admissions and have an overall mortality of 1%. Children of less than 5 years constitute about 25% of the total. In the US 30% are accidental and 40% self destructive. Ethyl alcohol ingestion is associated with 40% of all cases and multi-drug administration is common. In the UK helpful advice on treatment can be obtained 'round the clock' from the five National Poisons Information Centres.

Recognition and history

General supportive measures such as airway, O_2 therapy and intravenous fluids are continued during assessment of the patient. Most homes have to hand at least 20 potent pharmaceutical preparations and a variety of noxious chemicals such as weed killers and caustics. The scope for poisoning is thus enormous, and relatives can provide information as to the likely compound that has been administered. Often the patient has been receiving medication via the general practitioner so he should be questioned on this and other aspects of the medical history which might be relevant to treatment. Poisoning from drugs such as paracetamol demand urgent therapy, especially when there has been a delay in transfer to hospital, so this information should be obtained expeditiously.

Physical examination

Firstly, note additional injuries which may have been sustained as a result of the poisoning. A systematic review is necessary so that vital clues as to the cause and effect of poisoning are not missed.

(1) *Skin*
Pallor, cyanosis and clammy 'feel' suggest serious cardiovascular and respiratory compromise requiring urgent resuscitation prior to further examination. Bullae over pressure areas are characteristic of barbiturate poisoning whilst injection sites and scarring in the antecubital fossae suggest a history of drug abuse. Many drugs, such as organic insecticides are absorbed through the skin, so thorough cleaning and removal of contaminants has priority at this stage.

(2) *Neurological state*
Localising signs are very unusual in poisoning and suggest vascular or traumatic pathology necessitating computerised tomography. A simple 4 point scale is useful to describe the overall reaction of the patient:

I Drowsy, but responds to commands
II Responds appropriately to painful stimuli but not to command
III Only minimal response to maximal painful stimuli
IV Unresponsive

Cases in IV or those that are deteriorating rapidly need extra care for airway protection, oxygenation and CO_2 retention. Early intubation

and ventilation (IPPV) may become necessary. Pupillary size and reactivity are assessed, e.g. opiates give rise to pin-point pupils which enlarge following naloxone. Nystagmus suggests the possibility of Wernicke's encephalopathy.

(3) *Cardiorespiratory*
At all stages a close eye should be kept on the patient's circulation and respiration and appropriate supportive measures taken as and when necessary.

(4) *Other*
Other causes of unconsciousness should always be considered and investigated, e.g. postictal, diabetic or uraemic coma, myxoedema, stroke and so on.

Laboratory investigations

The Poisons Information centres provide useful advice on types and timing of samples necessary to provide a diagnosis or to assist management. This usually means gastric, urine and blood samples. Analysis and detection methods include paper chromatography, high performance liquid chromatography and mass spectrometry. Levels obtained and the potential for toxicity must be interpreted in the light of concurrent drugs administered (especially alcohol), the age of the patient and past medical history. They also provide a guide to the requirement of more invasive treatments such as haemodialysis and haemoperfusion.

Treatment

(1) *Supportive*
As mentioned above, attention is directed towards requirement for cardiorespiratory support at short notice. The frequency of hypoglycaemia, alcohol and opiates as a cause of 'coma' has led some units routinely to administer 50% glucose, naloxone and vitamin B complex intravenously, prior to definitive diagnosis.

(2) *Prevent further absorption of poisons*
In medical practice generally, drug absorption is a dynamic event, and is usually only partially

complete on the patient's arrival at hospital. Prevention of further absorption is of obvious importance and is approached in a variety of ways:

Remove from cause: this particularly applies to gas and smoke poisoning.
Gastric lavage: following ingestion of poisons, gastric motility is frequently markedly depressed, particularly following tricyclics, atropine-like compounds and opiates. Significant quantities of drug can be recovered by lavage, however, note that the technique is not without risk. It should never be carried out if caustics or long-chain hydrocarbons have been ingested as lavage can result in perforation and aspiration pneumonitis. The latter is likely if the patient has depressed airway reflexes; if in doubt the airway should be protected. The technique is carried out with the patient in the left lateral position, head down to prevent drug being pushed through the pylorus and into the small bowel, where further absorption will take place.
Emetics: in children, syrup of ipecacuanha (15–30 ml with orange juice) produces vomiting in 80% of patients in 5–10 minutes. Apomorphine is no longer recommended in the UK.
Catharsis: is rarely useful except in paraquat poisoning.
Adsorption: activated charcoal is a reliable non-specific adsorber of a variety of poisons, but to be effective it must be administered in a 10:1 ratio, so drugs such as paracetamol (500 mg, therefore 5 g charcoal per tablet) are less affected than imipramine (25 mg, therefore only 250 mg charcoal per tablet). It is usually administered following lavage, unless more specific agents are necessary.

(3) *Hasten elimination*
Internal: the human body is well equipped to detoxify most poisons provided cardiac output and oxygenation are sufficient to optimise liver function. It is clear that the hypotensive, hypercarbic and hypoxic patient has very little drug-metabolising ability. To prevent tubular reabsorption of non-ionised weak acids from the renal tubules back into the blood stream, the urine is alkalinised (with intravenous sodium bicarbonate) to change the drug into the non-transferable ionised form, e.g. salicylates. The opposite occurs with weak acids.
External: peritoneal and haemodialysis, haemoperfusion and exchange transfusion (in babies) are all employed when it is clear that drug levels are too high to rely on the body's own detoxification processes to be effective.

(4) *Antidotes*
A number of drug actions may be 'reversed' by the administration of antidotes some of which are mentioned below:

Naloxone: opiates and opioids
Doxapram: barbiturates (use not widely supported)
Physostigmine: tricyclics, benzodiazepines and anticholinergics
Antibodies: digoxin
Methionine and acetylcysteine: paracetamol
Desferrioxamine, calcium sodium edetate: iron and lead
Atropine and pralidoxime: organophosphorus insecticides
Cobalt edetate: cyanide

Specific poisons

The following are poisons which are commonly encountered in the accident and emergency department, only a broad outline of toxicity and treatment are included here.

(1) *Salicylates*
These cause allergy, bronchospasm and localised (gut) and generalised bleeding diatheses in susceptible subjects in normal dosage. Excessive ingestion (overdose or therapeutic in rheumatoid arthritis) leads to central stimulation with respiratory alkalosis, metabolic acidosis and hyperthermia. Gastric lavage and adsorption with charcoal is employed together with an alkaline diuresis. The latter involves large-scale fluid administration and the potential for circulatory overload and potassium loss, so fluid and electrolyte status must be closely observed.

(2) *Paracetamol*

Metabolism in the liver (if 5–10 g ingested) leads to free radical formation in excess of that which can be dealt with by sulphydryl (-SH) acceptors such as glutathione. The net result is a usually fatal hepatic necrosis. Lavage and adsorption followed by exogenous administration of -SH donors such as oral methionine or intravenous *N*-acetylcysteine, if paracetamol levels are excessive, is effective prevention if given early enough.

(3) *Alcohols*

Ethanol is not usually fatal in overdose but it does potentiate the actions of other depressants such as barbiturates. Methyl alcohol on the other hand is very toxic due to the formation of formic acid. (Methylated spirit contains 95% ethanol and 5% methanol.) Ethylene glycol (antifreeze) is metabolised to oxalates which chelate calcium and cause CNS and renal toxicity. Vitamin B complex should be administered to circumvent the possibility of Wernicke's encephalopathy in any comatose patient with a history of alcohol abuse.

(4) *Paraquat*

The paraquat in weedkiller is now combined with an emetic. Overdose causes delayed hepatic and pulmonary toxicity for which there is no specific treatment.

(5) *Barbiturates and benzodiazepines*

Supportive therapy only is required; in the former, high drug levels may necessitate haemodialysis or haemoperfusion.

(6) *Opiates and opioids*

These cause profound respiratory and cardiovascular depression with pin-point pupils. Pulmonary oedema and aspiration pneumonitis are common accompaniments. Supportive therapy and specific treatment with naloxone in repeated doses is indicated.

(7) *Tricyclic antidepressants*

Lavage and adsorption may be carried out even at a late stage as these drugs delay gastric emptying. They produce particularly cardiovascular and central nervous systems toxicity with hypotension, dysrhythmias and coma. The latter can be specifically reversed with physostigmine.

(8) *Cardiac drugs*

Include digoxin, beta blockers, calcium antagonists and antihypertensives. Overdose is managed pharmacologically, e.g. isoprenaline and glucagon with beta blockade, although specific antibodies have been useful in the treatment of digoxin overdose.

(9) *Carbon monoxide*

This is not present in household gas, except with incomplete combustion, but is frequently seen in association with burn injury and suicide attempts using car exhaust fumes in a confined space. It produces histotoxic anoxia as it binds much more avidly to haemoglobin than does oxygen. Treatment is with high concentrations of oxygen at ambient or hyperbaric pressures.

(10) *Heavy metals*

These are treated with chelating agents (as mentioned) following stomach lavage.

17

Chronic pain; approaches to management

Introduction

The sensation of pain is transduced at the periphery by three types of nerve endings called nociceptors; mechanoreceptors, thermoreceptors and polymodal receptors. The latter are the most important, and as their name suggests they may respond to any stimulus provided it is strong enough and thereby produce the sensation of pain. Impulses travel in the A delta and C fibres in the sensory nerves to the dorsal horn of the spinal cord. Here they may synapse in laminae 1–3, the marginal layer, decussate and then pass up the contralateral spinothalamic tract, or they may synapse in lamina 5 with the visceral pain afferents (thus providing an anatomical basis for referred pain) and pass up the ipsilateral anterior spinothalamic tract to the thalamus and cortex. The chemical transmitter in the laminae is substance P, and its release may be pre-synaptically inhibited by a descending pathway originating in the periaqueductal and the periventricular grey matter areas of the brain stem. Inhibition is mediated by the release of enkephalin, an opioid peptide which, like the endorphins, is derived from the parent molecule, opiocorticotropin.

This central pain inhibitory pathway possibly mediates the influence that changes in mentation, mood, anxiety state and so on can have on the perception of pain. The presence of naturally occurring morphine-like neurotransmitters (enkephalins and endorphins) provides an explanation for the actions of opiate analgesics.

Definition and Rationale of Chronic Pain

Chronic pain is distinguished from acute pain simply on the basis of duration, with a tendency to become more severe and incapacitating with time. If treated inadequately or too late, a vicious circle of debility leading to lowering of pain threshold and worsening of appreciation of pain may be set up. Pain stops serving the useful purpose of limiting movement of injured parts; itself becoming the disease rather than just a symptom.

The anaesthetist plays an important role in the management of these patients because of his special skills with nerve blockade, intra- and extradural analgesia, and knowledge of opiate pharmacology. Pain clinics have now been set up in many teaching and regional hospitals, usually staffed and managed by anaesthetists. Patients presenting to a pain clinic are always referred from other hospital departments or by general practitioners. Often they have been seen by several specialists and given little hope of improvement.

It is important to realise that pain causation is multifactorial. Even after being referred to the pain clinic, the treatment will frequently require the additional service of a neurologist, psychiatrist, orthopaedic and neurological surgeon.

The pain clinician is well aware of the role and pharmacology of a wide variety of adjuvant drugs such as non-steroidal analgesics (NSAIDS), antidepressants, anticonvulsants, chemotherapeutic agents, sedatives and tran-quillisers.

Diagnosis

A thorough, accurate history and physical examination are mandatory. Unnecessary suffering and perpetuation of a vicious circle must be avoided at an early stage and the confidence of the patient regained. Organic, treatable causes have usually been previously excluded by the referral clinician, but it must be confirmed independently by the pain clinician.

Types of Chronic Pain and their Treatment

Chronic pain syndromes fall into two broad categories, non-malignant chronic pain and malignant chronic pain.

(a) Non-malignant

(1) *The sympathetic dystrophies*
These may be divided into two main groups, reflex sympathetic dystrophy and causalgia. They are similar in origin, showing an increase in tonic activity of the sympathetic nervous system. Ischaemia leading to the release of pain modulating substances such as bradykinin and prostaglandins seems to be the mechanism. They occur in limbs and usually follow trauma or surgery, but may occur spontaneously as part of Raynaud's phenomenon in the upper limb. Typically, the initial pain of surgery fails to improve within a few days and is followed by hyperaesthesia, hyperhydrosis, muscle weakness and vasomotor disturbances. The latter may result in alternating constricted mottled skin with erythematous dilated skin. If not treated at this early stage, pain, muscle weakness and paraesthesia lead to loss of function, joint stiffness and fibrosis.

Causalgia is distinguished from reflex sympathetic dystrophy by the presence of an organic nerve lesion, such as in the median or the sciatic nerves, with direct involvement of the sympathetic fibres. The initial treatment consists of sympathetic block with bupivacaine to establish the diagnosis, followed by intravenous regional guanethidine or ketanserin. Alternatively or as an adjuvant, transcutaneous nerve stimulation (TCNS) may be used. It is imperative that the syndrome is immediately recognised by the surgeon or general practitioner and the patient referred for early treatment. Once the process is established, pain and loss of function may be permanent.

(2) *Lumbosacral and leg pain*
This constitutes the major category of chronic pain in the United Kingdom. It is usually due to nerve root inflammation and/or compression at the level of the intervertebral foramen. It follows injury or chronic degeneration of the intervertebral joint space and its characteristics vary according to the site of the lesion. Low back, buttock and thigh pain correspond to the 4th lumbar segment; pain which may extend to the heel involves the first sacral segment. The pain is made worse by exercise and attempted stretching of the nerve (e.g. straight leg raising). If the pain and loss of function are progressive and affect autonomic function such as bladder emptying, then the patient must be referred to a neurologist for expert advice.

Treatment consists of bed rest supplemented with NSAIDS, but should the condition not improve, epidural injection of a mixture of pred-nisolone and bupivacaine is the treatment of choice. This is accompanied by passive leg straightening (sometimes under general anaesthesia) which stretches the nerve roots to aid steroid penetration. It is important that the extent of the disability with regard to pain, loss of function, sensory deficit and reflex loss is carefully documented, as repeated injections may be necessary; the progression of the condition under treatment is usually unpredictable.

Other causes of pain in the back and lower limb are facet or sacroiliac disease and myofasciitis. The former may follow torsion injury and if severe may be relieved by facet block with bupivacaine. The latter are distinguished from nerve entrapment by the presence of 'trigger points' which when compressed or electrically stimulated mimic the pain; when injected with local analgesics there is instantaneous relief.

(3) *Cervical and upper limb pain*

These follow the same pattern as the lower limb, with pain and disability reflecting the nerve roots involved by trauma or degenerative disease. Upper cervical lesions produce vague headaches, and lower lesions will involve the hand with pain, paraesthesiae and loss of function. Treatment is initially conservative with collars and NSAIDS. Resistant cases may need cervical epidural injection and transcutaneous nerve stimulation.

(4) *Peripheral neuropathies and herpetic neuralgia*

There are many causes of peripheral neuropathy which produce a painful neuralgia, the commonest being the nerve entrapment syndrome. This may appear spontaneously or following excessive pressure or surgery. The latter may involve cutting a nerve route with the resultant 'neuroma' being trapped in scar tissue, e.g. post-thoracotomy pain.

Pain associated with acute herpetic lesions often progresses, particularly in the elderly, to continued pain long after the herpetic lesions have healed. It is becoming increasingly evident that early and adequate treatment of the acute pain with analgesics and/or sympathetic block will significantly reduce the incidence of this unpleasant condition. In the established case transcutaneous nerve stimulation complemented with phenothiazines or antidepressant drugs may be required.

Trigeminal neuralgia is one of the most unpleasant of pain syndromes, and does not respond to conventional analgesics. Treatment consists of carbamazepine (an anti-epileptic agent) followed if necessary by chemical trigeminal ganglionectomy.

(5) *Phantom limb pain*

Postamputation phantom limb pain is extremely problematical and requires combined therapy with analgesics, psychotropic drugs, nerve blocks and transcutaneous nerve stimulation.

The severity of the syndrome is related to the degree of pain suffered previous to amputation. There is sympathetic nervous system involvement; some patients respond with a prolonged remission after a single sympathetic block with bupivacaine.

(b) Malignant chronic pain

It is important to realise that pain occurs in two-thirds of patients with advanced cancer, but in one-third of these pain is not due to the growth itself. In these cases, appropriate treatment is as outlined under non-malignant chronic pain. It is very important to realise that cancer is a disease which has implications for the patient as a whole, so the pain must be treated with this in mind. Thus, anxiety, depression, insomnia and poor appetite which are experienced by the majority of cancer patients at some stage of their illness must all be treated in addition to the use of powerful opiates.

The necessity to make an accurate diagnosis of the cause of pain must be emphasised, such as between nerve compression and destruction. In the former analgesics, steroids and nerve blocks are usually effective, whilst in the latter they are virtually useless, and more appropriate therapy will include psychotropic drugs. Also, it is in this field that adjuvant therapy, apart from pure analgesia is so useful. For instance, muscle spasm is treated with baclofen; raised intracranial pressure headache with steroids and diuretics; stabbing type pains with anticonvulsants, and so on. Relief of symptoms such as these which are associated with cancer pain may serve to raise the patient's pain threshold and make specific analgesic therapy more effective.

Pain-relieving drugs must be prescribed rationally, starting with simple NSAIDS such as aspirin or paracetamol, progressing via mild opiates such as codeine to strong opiates such as morphine. Combination of aspirin with codeine and paracetamol may obviate the need for early introduction of the stronger morphine. The latter is given orally to allow the patient greater freedom and comfort, and must be given regularly to prevent pain breakthrough. The addition of a phenothiazine reduces nausea and vomiting during the early stages of treatment in the ambulant patient and may also potentiate the analgesia. Respiratory depression and addiction are minor problems in cancer patients. In resistant cases more heroic measures such as pituitary ablation (e.g. breast cancer), dorsal root entry zone cordotomy and intrathecal phenol may be used, but the risks associated with these techniques restricts their use to terminal malignant conditions.

18

Techniques in regional analgesia

Regional blocks should be carried out with resuscitation equipment and expertise immediately available. A few of the relatively safe and easy blocks, which have a high rate of success, will be described. Intravenous regional anaesthesia is discussed with emphasis on its complications.

In addition, the technique of epidural and spinal anaesthesia (which should only be performed by the specialist) will be outlined, as they are often the method of choice for surgery.

Intercostal Nerve Blocks

Indications

Few therapeutic measures cause as much gratitude in the patient as intercostal nerve blocks following rib fractures. It is also a very useful block to follow the insertion of a chest drain; the pain of a subcostal incision for cholecystectomy is also greatly relieved by blocking the 6th to 11th right intercostal nerves. Postherpetic neuralgia may be greatly helped with repeated blocks with bupivacaine mixed with prednisolone (Chapter 17).

Preparation

Intercostal nerve blocks can be done with the patient sitting or lying on the side.

Bupivacaine is the anaesthetic of choice because of its prolonged action. A 20 ml syringe is filled with anaesthetic and a 21G (green) or 23G (blue) needle attached.

The operator should scrub the hands or wear sterile gloves, and prepare the skin with an antiseptic solution.

Technique

Intercostal nerves are best blocked at the angle of the rib which ensures that the lateral cutaneous branch is included in the block. The rib is felt 7–9 cm from the mid-line by palpation with the 2nd and 3rd fingers of the left hand, and the needle inserted through the skin, pointing cephalad (as shown in Fig. 18.1(a)), until it meets the bone which gives an unmistakable inelastic feeling of hitting hard wood. Then the needle is withdrawn a few mm and advanced in a more caudal direction until it meets the rib again. This procedure is repeated a few times until no bone is felt; at this point the needle should be advanced a further 3 mm through a layer giving an elastic feeling; this is usually accompanied by a sudden 'give' or 'pop' as the needle enters the sheath of the neurovascular bundle running along the lower edge of the rib. At this point 3–4 ml of bupivacaine should be injected, after aspiration to ensure that the needle is not in a blood vessel. The injection of this volume should feel very easy since the anaesthetic is going into the loose tissue surrounding the neurovascular bundle, as seen in Fig. 18.1(b). The needle should not be advanced any further as there is a risk of entering the pleural cavity.

The block is then repeated at other intercostal spaces as necessary, but the total amount of 20 ml of 0.5% bupivacaine (100 mg) must not be exceeded (in the 70 kg patient). Systemic

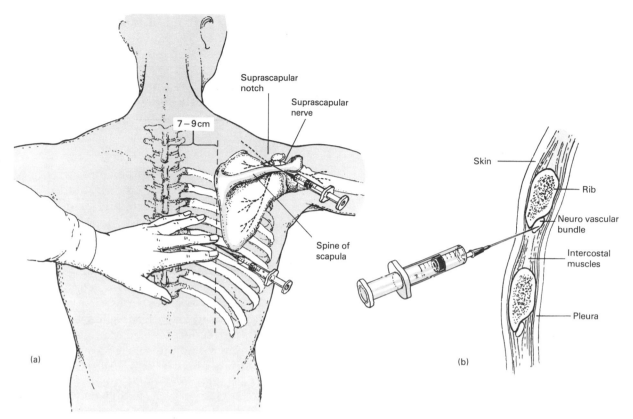

Fig. 18.1 Suprascapular and intercostal nerve blocks. (a) Landmarks and position of syringes to perform blocks. (b) Cross section of the thoracic wall to show position of the neurovascular bundle, and angle of approach with the needle for intercostal nerve block

absorption of anaesthetic is very rapid after intercostal block, so great care must be taken not to exceed the maximum total dose (Chapter 5). Pain relief usually lasts up to 12 hours, at which time the block may be repeated.

Suprascapular Nerve Block

This block is very simple and safe to perform, and provides rewarding relief of shoulder pain (e.g. after trauma or after manipulation or reduction of dislocated shoulder under general anaesthesia).

It is best done with the patient sitting; the spine of the scapula is palpated and its mid point marked on the skin with a pen. A long (6 cm or more) 21 or 23G needle is inserted through the skin one finger width above the pen

mark, pointing slightly medially and downwards, until the bone of the supraspinatus fossa is met. This should be very close to the suprascapular notch where the suprascapular nerve passes (see Fig. 18.1(a)). Paraesthesia, experienced as pain at the tip of the shoulder, may sometimes be elicited. At this point 5–10 ml of 0.5% bupivacaine is injected, after pulling on the plunger of the syringe to ensure that the tip does not lie in a blood vessel. Analgesia of the shoulder should last for up to 10–12 hours.

Ring Block of the Finger or Toe

Fingers and toes are supplied by two dorsal and two palmar (or plantar) nerves. These can be blocked effectively for minor surgical procedures. A fine 25G (orange) needle should be used; after preparation of the skin the needle

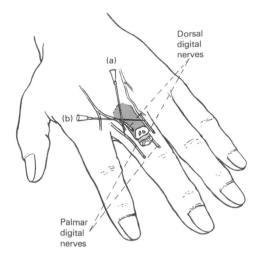

Fig. 18.2 Ring block of the third digit of the left hand. (a) Position of 25G needle to block lateral dorsal and palmar branches. (b) Needle turned horizontally and reinserted to infiltrate dorsal aspect of the skin. Once this is completed, the needle may be inserted medially, parallel to (a), to block the medial branches

is inserted dorsally at one side of the base of the finger (or toe) and advanced close to the surface of the bone until its tip lies close to the palmar (or plantar) surface. Then, while slowly withdrawing the needle, inject 2–3 ml 2% plain lignocaine.

Before the needle is totally withdrawn, it should be deflected and advanced to the other side and a further 0.5–1 ml injected under the skin at the point where the needle is to be reinserted to block the digital nerves on the other side of the finger. Figure 18.2 sketches this procedure.

The injection of anaesthetic must be done slowly because the distension of the tissues in this region is very painful. Note that adrenaline or other vasoconstrictors must NOT be used in this block.

Intravenous Regional Analgesia of the Arm (Bier's Block)

It cannot be emphasised enough that this block must NOT, under any circumstances be undertaken without having full resuscitation facilities

and expertise at hand. It should be noted that, if the dose of local anaesthetic injected i.v. for the procedure should gain rapid access into the systemic circulation, it will produce toxic side effects ranging from convulsions to a state of general anaesthesia with respiratory and cardiovascular depression.

Preparation

The patient should lie supine and comfortably, with the affected arm supported by a side board. A cannula should be inserted in the dorsum of the opposite hand for easy access to a vein should toxic effects occur. It is sometimes advisable to sedate the patient with a small intravenous dose of a benzodiazepine (e.g. 5–10 mg diazepam) just prior to the injection of local anaesthetic in the other arm. A suitable tourniquet (type used for orthopaedic surgery of the arm, or a specially devised double cuff tourniquet) is put round the affected arm over cotton wool padding, and carefully secured to prevent accidental deflation or detachment.

Technique

A 20 or 22G cannula is then inserted into a vein of the dorsum of the hand (if this location interferes with surgery or is inconvenient, it may be inserted into any other superficial vein of the arm as distally as possible), and the arm raised vertically for three minutes, to reduce the volume of blood contained within the venous compartment. If the lesion to be treated surgically is not painful, an Esmarch rubber bandage can be tightly applied round the whole limb, draining the blood away into the general circulation. If the bandage cannot be applied, the brachial artery may be compressed with the fingers (without obstructing venous return) for 30 seconds while keeping the arm upright, and the tourniquet inflated rapidly to 250 mmHg.

The pressure in the tourniquet must be carefully watched throughout the whole procedure and not allowed to drop. With the tourniquet inflated, 25–30 ml of 0.5% lignocaine is then injected very slowly through the cannula with the arm horizontal, watching for signs of vein distension (see Fig. 18.3). If veins appear distended, the rate of injection must be reduced

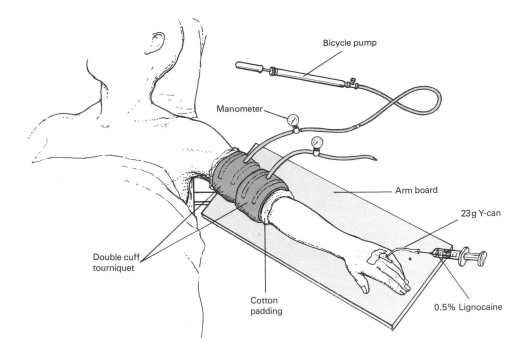

Fig. 18.3 Technique of intravenous regional analgesia (Bier's block)

or stopped, because pressures may be generated within the venous system sufficient to cause leakage of anaesthetic into the general circulation.

Paraesthesiae are soon felt by the patient, and within 5–10 minutes a complete sensory and motor block should ensue, lasting for as long as the tourniquet is applied (up to 1 hour). If a double cuffed tourniquet is used, the proximal cuff is first inflated. When analgesia of the arm is established, the distal cuff (lying on anaesthetised skin) is inflated to the same pressure and the proximal one deflated. This usually relieves the discomfort associated with the pressure of the cuff.

The tourniquet must not be let down for at least 15 minutes after the injection of the local anaesthetic. This time interval ensures that enough anaesthetic has diffused out of the vascular compartment, such that the amount entering the circulation as a 'bolus' is not sufficient to cause toxic effects.

Toxic reactions

Should the tourniquet be accidentally deflated less than 15 minutes after injection of lignocaine, the patient must be closely monitored for side effects; paraesthesiae of the tongue and lips is usually the first symptom of systemic overdose.

Should an epileptiform fit occur, 10 mg of diazepam should be injected intravenously through the butterfly needle in the opposite arm, and 100% oxygen given through a face mask until the convulsion is over. The dose of diazepam may be repeated twice if necessary, but it must be remembered that it will potentiate the respiratory depression caused by lignocaine. An intravenous infusion should be set up in the 'free' arm.

The first toxic symptom may be loss of consciousness. If respiratory depression occurs (also following a convulsion) manual ventilation with 100% oxygen must be started immediately and monitoring of pulse, blood pressure and ECG instituted. The P-Q interval of the ECG is likely

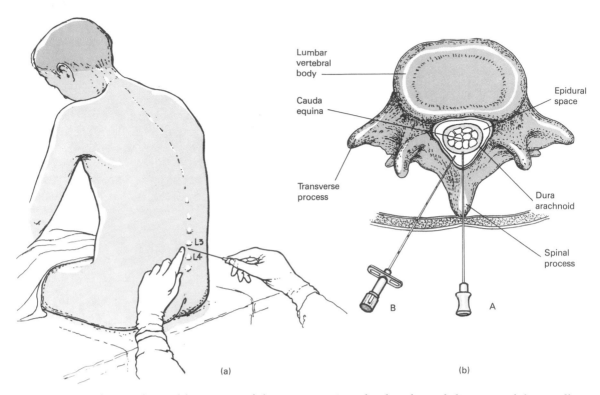

Fig. 18.4 Spinal anaesthesia (a) Position of the sitting patient, landmarks and direction of the needle. (b) Horizontal section of a lumbar intervertebral space to show the position of the tip of the needle for sub-arachnoid (A) and extradural (B) anaesthesia

to be prolonged, the heart rate slow, and the blood pressure low. If systolic pressure is below 60 mmHg, 3–5 mg boluses of ephedrine may be given intravenously (up to 30 mg total). If the blood pressure is unrecordable (no pulses felt in the carotids) external cardiac massage must be started (Chapter 14).

Epidural and Subarachnoid Blocks

Epidurals may be performed at any level of the thoracic, lumbar or sacral spine. Lumbar epidurals at L2-3 or L3-4 level are the commonest, followed by the sacral or caudal approach. Lumbar epidural or subarachnoid blocks are suitable for most surgery of the lower abdomen and lower limbs. Epidural analgesia is also very useful for the relief of post-operative and labour pains.

Both are effective firstly upon the sympathetic, and then upon the sensory and motor fibres. The sympathetic blockade always causes vasodilatation in the lower half of the body and a fall in blood pressure. An intravenous infusion must therefore be set up beforehand, to treat this almost certain complication.

(a) Epidurals

The anaesthetic solution is injected into the epidural space, composed of loose connective tissue and veins, which surrounds the dura in the spinal canal (Fig. 18.4). Volumes ranging from 8 ml of 0.5% bupivacaine (for relief of pain in labour or post-operatively) to 30 ml of 0.5% bupivacaine or 1.5% lignocaine (for lower abdominal or hip surgery) may be injected directly through a needle or through a fine plastic catheter. The plastic catheter has the advantage of allowing top-ups if left in situ (usually 2–3 cm inside the epidural space).

Note that the higher doses are close to those causing systemic side effects. Once the anaesthetic is injected, it will take from 20 minutes (1.5% lignocaine) to 40 minutes (0.5% bupivacaine) to establish the sensory block, which then lasts up to 90 minutes with bupivacaine. Occasionally the block produced is unsatisfactory for surgery because one side or a particular segment remains resistant to the effect of the drug regardless of repeated top-ups or repositioning of the catheter.

Caudals are a form of epidural analgesia, but the epidural space is reached through the sacrococcygeal membrane. The nature, rate and seriousness of complications is the same as in lumbar epidurals. Single-shot caudals with 0.5% bupivacaine are often given for post-operative pain relief after perineal surgery (e.g. circumcision in children).

Top-ups

Topping up epidurals through the indwelling catheter carries identical risks to the initial administration. The risk of injecting the wrong drug is always present, and it cannot be emphasised enough that only specially trained personnel, fully aware of the possible complications, should perform this technique. It is often done by specially trained midwives in labour wards; the blood pressure must be monitored at 5 minute intervals for 20 minutes after topping-up. A well-drilled routine should be established to deal with complications such as precipitous fall in blood pressure or total paralysis.

(b) Subarachnoid (spinal) analgesia

The subarachnoid space is reached with a fine needle (22 or 25G) as if for a diagnostic lumbar puncture (Fig. 18.4). The correct position of the tip of the needle is confirmed by obtaining clear CSF dripping off the hub. Only 1–2 ml of anaesthetic is injected to produce a block equivalent to that obtained with 20–30 ml in the epidural space, the effect being obtained within 5–10 minutes.

Subarachnoid analgesia is very reliable in its effects; patchy blocks are very rare, an advantage over epidurals. It is however a single-shot procedure; top-ups are not usually possible. A percentage of patients, varying from 1 to 3%, complain of headaches post-operatively due to leakage of CSF through the hole made by the needle in the dura. The incidence is lowest with fine 25G needles. The anaesthetic solutions used are normally mixed with 6–9% dextrose to become hyperbaric (heavier, or more dense than CSF), such that by positioning the patient appropriately a more regionalised block (e.g. one-sided) may be obtained.

The most commonly used anaesthetic solutions are: heavy cinchocaine (Nupercaine, Dibucaine) 0.5% in 6% dextrose; heavy mepivacaine (Carbocaine) 4% in 5% dextrose; and heavy bupivacaine (Marcaine) 0.5% in 8% dextrose.

Late complications of epidural and subarachnoid blockade may occur, such as persistent paraesthesia or weakness, often of a patchy nature. Their management is beyond the scope of this book.

Appendix A

Principles of pharmacology relevant to anaesthesia and intensive care

Only 25 years ago, the amount of information deemed necessary for efficient clinical use of a common drug would fit into a few lines of text. Approximately 500 new drugs have since been introduced for clinical use, and many more will be introduced in the future. Clinicians are now presented with much information on newly released drugs, including:

Theory of action,
Description of effects in normal and diseased states,
Plasma concentration – response relationships,
Absorption disposition and elimination,
Pharmacokinetics,
Interference with other drugs,
Effects of overdosage,
Storage, cost, etc.

Present standards of practice demand extensive knowledge of pharmacological principles. Anaesthesia provides excellent examples of the application of such principles.

Cell Membranes

All drugs need to cross at least one cell membrane to produce their desired effects. Factors affecting this process are:

Size and shape of drug molecules

These determine passage of drugs through pores in cell membranes, epithelia and endothelia. For example, confinement of plasma expanders to the vascular compartment depends on molecular size. Molecular configuration of drugs determine binding to specific cell surface proteins for active transport across the membrane. Active transport is highly selective, saturable, requires energy $(ATP \rightarrow ADP + P)$, and may operate against a concentration gradient (e.g. amino acids, iodine). If it does not operate against a gradient it is called facilitated diffusion (e.g. glucose).

Lipid solubility and ionisation

(1) *Lipid solubility*
This is the most important determinant of diffusibility across cell membranes because of the lipid nature of their constituents. Lipid-soluble drugs easily cross the blood–brain and placental barriers.

(2) *Ionisation*
Drugs with electrovalent bonds dissociate in aqueous solution as weak acids or weak bases. Acid drugs are maximally ionised at high pH, and basic drugs at low pH. Thus, the proportion of a drug in ionised form depends on the pH of the tissue or medium where it is

present. Because cell membranes are electrically charged, the permeability for the ionised portion of drug is much less than for the non-ionised portion. The latter is usually lipid soluble. For example, pancuronium, being largely ionised in plasma, does not cross the blood–brain and placental barriers. Weakly basic drugs, poorly ionised at plasma pH, may accumulate in the stomach after i.v. administration; this is due to passive diffusion into a medium with lower pH, where most of the drug ionises, thus preventing its diffusion back to plasma. The central analgesic fentanyl (a weak base) is such an example, being reabsorbed 2–3 hours later as the stomach contents pass into the intestine (at a higher pH). This effect is known as 'ion trapping'.

Absorption

Drugs may be given through a variety of routes. There is always some systemic distribution, even when drugs are applied topically.

(a) Gastrointestinal route

Lipid solubility and ionisation are important in absorption (see above). Drugs given orally are absorbed into portal blood and pass through the liver before reaching the general circulation. Often, this 'first pass' through the liver causes a large reduction in the amount of drug available (e.g. propranolol). Sublingual or rectal application obviate this effect. Bioavailability is the percentage of an oral dose reaching the systemic circulation; it is determined by absorption and first pass metabolism.

(b) Injection

Intravenous injection produces a peak plasma concentration within one circulation time (approximately one minute). In terms of effects it is the most predictable route and the one used in emergencies. Intramuscular and subcutaneous injections are variably absorbed depending on local blood perfusion.

(c) Mucous membranes

Skin, conjunctivae, nasal and other mucosae are examples of routes for topical application, often leading to sufficient systemic absorption to produce general effects. For example, plasma pseudocholinesterase may be inhibited by ecothiopate eye drops thus prolonging the effects of suxamethonium.

(d) Inhalation of gases, vapours or droplets

Finely dispersed droplets of salbutamol or steroids are commonly self-administered in the treatment of bronchospasm. Of more specific interest in this context is the administration of inhalational anaesthetics. These are given with the purpose of producing an effect upon the brain; the rapidity of this effect depends upon factors discussed in Chapter 5.

Distribution and Elimination

Drugs are not evenly distributed throughout all tissues of the body. A proportion may bind to plasma proteins; well-perfused tissues such as the brain may initially be exposed to higher concentrations of drug before redistribution to other tissues. Breakdown or excretion may be so fast that equilibrium is never reached.

Phamacokinetics is concerned with time-dependent changes in plasma concentration following administration of drugs (also described as 'what the patient does to the drug'). Knowledge of three pharmacokinetic parameters (clearance, half-life and volume of distribution) is very useful to obtain optimum results for drugs with a narrow margin between toxic and therapeutic effects.

Pharmacokinetic characteristics of drugs

Most studies of drug kinetics refer only to profiles of plasma concentration following intravenous injection. Fortunately, most drug effects are closely related to plasma concentrations.

After single injection, plasma levels decline according to well-defined patterns. Abstract models representing one or more 'compartments' are frequently used to help predict duration of effects.

(1) *Single compartment model*

In this model, the plot of plasma concentration (following single bolus i.v. injection) against time is a simple exponential curve, which appears as a straight line if the logarithm of concentration is taken (Fig. A.1). This is called first order kinetics, in which a constant fraction of drug present in plasma is eliminated per unit of time. Many drugs in current use show this pattern of distribution and elimination.

The volume of distribution (Vd) can be calculated by dividing the dose injected (D) by the estimated initial plasma concentration (Ci), obtained by extrapolating the straight line in Fig. A.1):

$$Vd = D/Ci$$

Drugs remaining within the vascular compartment, such as dextran 70, have a Vd around 5 litres. Drugs highly bound to tissues, such as lignocaine, may have a Vd exceeding 60 litres.

Plasma half-life of a drug ($t_{1/2}$) is the time taken for plasma concentration to be halved. It may be measured directly from the elimination curve.

Clearance (Cl) is the volume of plasma completely cleared of drug per unit of time, and can be calculated as follows:

$$Cl = 0.69 \times Vd/(t_{1/2}) \quad \text{in ml min}^{-1}$$

Clearance is the best measure of elimination capacity of the body, and is very useful for clinical comparisons. These three parameters may be used for therapeutic purposes, such as deciding upon loading and maintenance doses.

Steady-state concentrations in plasma (Css) may be achieved by means of continuous i.v. infusions (e.g. lignocaine), when the rate of drug elimination equals the rate of administration:

$$Css = \text{Infusion Rate}/\text{Clearance}$$

If the drug is administered as boluses (or tablets) at regular intervals, the plasma levels fluctuate, but the 'average' steady-state concentration (Ca) can be calculated as follows:

$$Ca = (Dm \times F)/(Ti \times Cl)$$

where Dm is the maintenance dose, Ti the dosing interval and F the bioavailability if administered by the oral route. If the drug is started at the maintenace dosage it takes 4 half-lives to reach 94% of the steady-state plasma concentration.

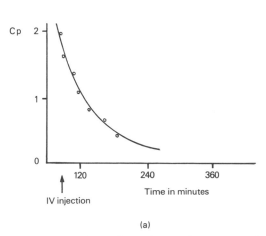

(a)

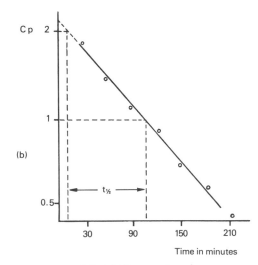

(b)

Fig. A.1 Example of first order kinetics (single compartment model) (a) Plasma drug concentration (Cp), against time, following intravenous bolus injection (linear scale). (b) The same as in (a), plotted in a semilogarithmic scale; $t_{1/2}$ is the half-life. Cp units are arbitrary

Sometimes it is important to bring plasma concentration to steady-state therapeutic levels in less time; a loading dose (Dl) may be administered,

Dl = Css × Vd

or   Dl = (Dm × $t_{1/2}$)/(Ti × 0.693)

followed by regular administration of a maintenance dose. The above calculations apply to drugs eliminated by first order processes, and the units used (e.g. mg, ml, minute) must be consistent between equations.

Example of calculation of loading and maintenance doses for lignocaine:

Desirable steady state level in plasma:
Css = 2 mgl^{-1}
Volume of distribution:
Vd = 1100 ml kg^{-1} or 77 l (70 kg man)
Clearance:
Cl = 9.2 ml min^{-1} kg^{-1} or 0.64 l min^{-1} (70 kg man)
Calculation of loading dose:

Dl = Css × Vd   or   2 × 77
   = 154 mg

Calculation of maintenance dose:

Dm = Css × Cl   or   2 × 0.64
   = 1.3 mg min^{-1}

Thus, the volume of distribution determines the loading dose and the clearance determines the maintenance dose. This is important for drugs principally excreted via the kidney, when administered to patients in renal failure. Loading dose will be the same or even higher than in patients with normal renal function, as Vd may be increased. Maintenace dose, however, will be markedly reduced (lower doses or longer dose intervals) in view of the much lower drug clearance.

(2) *Two compartment model*
After bolus i.v. injection into a 'central compartment', many drugs exhibit a short therapeutic effect because they are rapidly distributed into 'peripheral compartments', such as visceral organs with high blood supply. Drugs falling within this pattern of disposition are sometimes described as 'short-acting' because

of the rapid fall in plasma concentration during the distribution phase, e.g. thiopentone and fentanyl. They have 'cumulative' effects if administered repeatedly, due to slower elimination from the 'peripheral' compartments. There are thus two half-lives to consider, $t_{1/2}$ distribution and $t_{1/2}$ elimination.

(3) *Zero order kinetics*
A few drugs follow a quite different pattern of elimination (e.g. phenytoin, ethanol and thiopentone in high doses). Above a certain plasma level a constant amount of drug is eliminated per unit of time, regardless of plasma concentration. This is attributed to saturation of metabolic processes. Below saturation level, first order kinetics apply.

Drug elimination

The patterns of elimination described above are the result of chemical alteration and/or excretion of the drug.

(1) *Chemical alteration*
Chemical alteration or biotransformation is carried out mainly in the liver, and therefore is dependent upon liver blood flow. Blood levels of orally administered drugs which undergo substantial 'first pass' metabolism, such as morphine and propranolol, are markedly increased if liver blood flow is reduced. This can cause toxicity. A few drugs (e.g. suxamethonium) are metabolised by plasma enzymes, and more rarely by enzyme systems in other organs, e.g. kidney or lung.

Biotransformation of active drugs in the liver may lead to breakdown products which are also active; for example diazepam is metabolised to desmethyldiazepam which is equipotent to diazepam, but with a $t_{1/2}$ elimination of 53 hours compared to 32 hours for diazepam. This is of importance in long-term administration. Pancuronium is also metabolised into active compounds. Some inactive drugs are metabolised into active ones (e.g. triclofos into trichloroethanol).

Biotransformation in the liver is carried out in a variety of ways broadly classified as synthetic and non-synthetic. Non-synthetic or phase I reactions are carried out by hepatic intracellular microsomal systems requiring NADPH, oxygen and cytochrome P-450. Examples are oxidation, reduction and hydrolysis.

Examples of synthetic, conjugation or phase II reactions are glucuronide formation, acetylation, sulphate conjugation, and methylation. Most reactions render lipid soluble drugs water soluble, facilitating renal excretion.

A few drugs are metabolised by a single process, but the majority are metabolised in two phases; firstly by a non-synthetic (phase I) reaction and secondly by a synthetic (phase II) reaction, each causing inactivation of the drug. Some of the above reactions, particularly microsomal oxidation and reduction, can be significantly enhanced by previous exposure to the same drug or to other drugs metabolised by the same microsomal system. This is called enzyme induction. Classic examples are the chronic intake of phenobarbitone or alcohol which increase tolerance to analgesics and anaesthetic agents.

Inhibition of enzymes occurs with drugs such as metronidazole, erythromycin and sulphonamides.

(2) Excretion

Excretion of unaltered drug or its metabolites occurs mainly in the kidney, but also through the bile (e.g. tubocurarine) or through the lung (inhalational anaesthetics). If the plasma kinetics are highly dependent upon the renal excretion of unmetabolised drug (e.g. gallamine, gentamicin), then the state of the renal function is important in determining duration of effect.

Mechanism of Drug Action (Pharmacodynamics)

Pharmacodynamics is the study of mechanisms of drug action (also described as 'what the drug does to the body'). Most drugs act upon receptors on the surface of cells in a highly specific fashion; very small modifications of the molecular structure of the drug may lead to a complete change of pharmacological activity. The study of this structure–activity relationship has led to the rational development of many new drugs in the past three decades.

A smaller proportion of drugs do not produce effects by interaction with specialised receptors. For example, the volatile anaesthetic agents are thought to act non-specifically upon the lipid component of cell membranes; magnesium sulphate exerts its purgative action by an osmotic effect within the gut; other drugs interfere with DNA, the genetic material.

(a) Receptors

Receptors are situated on the surface of cells, and mediate the action of natural chemical messengers upon intracellular mechanisms. The nature of transmitter–receptor interactions is not completely understood. The quantities of receptor molecules per gram of tissue is itself subject to complex regulation; e.g. thyroid hormone regulates the synthesis of beta receptors on heart cells.

The study of drug effects led to the discovery of different receptors naturally stimulated by the one transmitter; e.g. alpha and beta adrenergic receptors.

Drug–receptor interaction may be classified as agonist, partial agonist and competitive antagonist.

Agonists bind to the receptor initiating activity; they have affinity for that receptor, e.g. morphine binds to opiate receptors on the surface of neurons in the spinal cord.

Competitive antagonists also bind to receptors (have affinity) but do not initiate activity. They may displace agonists, e.g. naloxone has higher affinity for opiate receptors than morphine, displacing the latter at lower concentrations.

Partial agonists bind more avidly to receptors (have greater affinity) but are often less efficacious (have less activity than full agonists). In the presence of high concentrations of agonists a partial agonist will displace the first, thus acting like an antagonist. If the concentration of agonist is low, the effect of partial agonists is additive.

Note that the term 'receptor' may also appear in a physiological context referring to 'sensory receptors'; these are complex structures such as muscle spindles or retinal rods.

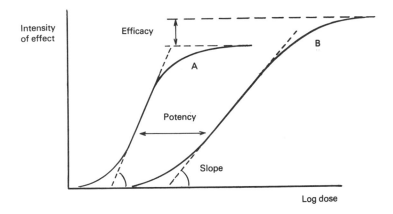

Fig. A.2 Log dose–effect relationship. Drug A is more potent than drug B, but less efficacious. Most drugs show an 'S' shaped relationship as in this graph

(b) Structure–activity relationship

The activity and other properties of many drugs are related to chemical structure. New drugs are 'tailored' to fit therapeutic requirements. For example enflurane was successfully designed to produce general anaesthesia based on the ether molecule, but with a lower solubility in blood, less irritant effects and non-flammability. Present day design of new antibacterial drugs is highly sophisticated.

(c) Pharmacodynamic characterisation

Many definitions fall within this general heading, such as potency, efficacy, therapeutic index, and tolerance. Some of the useful concepts are better understood with the help of Fig. A.2, depicting the usual sigmoid shape of the log dose or log concentration versus effect relationship. Not all drugs have a graded response; some drugs produce an all-or-none type of response, such as suppression of dysrhythmias; plots similar to Fig. A.2 may still be constructed but in terms of frequency of occurrence of therapeutic effect in a population of individuals.

(1) Potency is related to the concentration or dosage which produces an effect (also 'affinity', in receptor theory).
(2) Efficacy is the maximal possible response which can be produced (also 'activity', in receptor theory).

(3) Side effects are those produced in addition to the principal therapeutic effect.
(4) Therapeutic index or selectivity is the ratio between the dose producing undesired effects and the dose producing therapeutic effects.
(5) Tolerance is the decrease, over a period of time, in therapeutic effect produced by identical doses of the drug.
(6) Tachyphylaxis is the rapid development of tolerance.
(7) The median effective dose ED_{50} is that required to produce a certain intensity of effect in 50% of subjects.
(8) The median lethal dose LD_{50} is that which produces lethal effects in 50% of individuals (this evidently only applies to animal tests).

(d) Plasma levels

Plasma levels may now be measured for a large number of drugs. It is an expensive complement to drug therapy and should be used only if there are clear advantages. Blood samples must be taken at specified times after drug administration to be of any value. The indications are:

(1) In some cases of treatment failure when there is a predictable relationship between plasma concentration and effects, e.g. anticonvulsants.

(2) Use of drugs with a low therapeutic index or very serious side effects, e.g. gentamycin, theophylline.

(3) Serious drug interactions such as those occurring with warfarin.

(4) In suicidal or accidental overdosage, e.g. paracetamol levels determine the management policy.

Drug Interaction with Anaesthetic Agents

Caution about interaction of anaesthetic agents with other drugs is important. It may occur by competition for binding sites in plasma proteins, saturation of metabolic pathways in liver or plasma, inhibition of inactivating enzymes, or by physiological potentiation. Some of the best known examples are:

(a) Ecothiopate eye drops used in glaucoma inhibit plasma cholinesterase prolonging the effect of suxamethonium.

(b) Aminoglycoside antibiotics (e.g. gentamycin) have neuromuscular blocking properties of their own, potentiating the effect of pancuronium and other relaxants.

(c) Monoamine oxidase inhibitors (e.g. iproniazid), by altering the metabolism of catecholamines and central analgesics, cause some patients to respond unpredictably to morphine or pethidine with hypotension, hypertension or coma. Response to inotropes and hypotensive agents is also unpredictable.

Appendix B
Physiology and pharmacology of the autonomic nervous system

The concept of autonomic nervous system has resulted from anatomical and physiological studies carried out since Langley coined the term in 1898. Functionally it is defined as that part of the nervous system which regulates visceral functions, circulation, ventilation and temperature control. For this reason it has also been named the vegetative or involuntary nervous system.

It is a set of afferent and efferent nerve fibres and integrative neurons within the central nervous system constituting the anatomical basis of regulatory reflexes. Studies in the last 20 years have shown that some regulatory functions can obey volitional control, suggesting a cortical representation of the autonomic system. This is the foundation of 'bio-feedback' techniques, whereby a subject is helped in sensing the state of an autonomic function by a measuring device, e.g. a skin temperature probe or a blood pressure monitor.

The clinical importance of the regulatory functions is obvious. The great majority of drugs in common use are either specifically designed to modify autonomic functions or have serious side effects upon them.

Anatomy and Physiology

The first demonstration of the chemical nature of neurotransmission was made by Otto Loewi (1921) using the vagal innervation of the heart.

The concept of a drug receptor, as defined in the previous chapter, has also emerged from experimental work in autonomic structures, on finding that different drugs may mimic or block different effects of the same natural neurotransmitter at different end organs. Traditionally, the autonomic nervous system has been divided into two anatomically and functionally distinct efferent divisions: the sympathetic and the parasympathetic. Figure B.1 shows a schematic diagram of the anatomy and best-known neurotransmitters.

(a) Sympathetic system

This emerges from the thoracic and lumbar segments of the spinal cord (T1-L2), supplying the pre-ganglionic innervation of the para-vertebral chain of sympathetic ganglia and abdominal plexuses. Synaptic transmission in the ganglia is mainly cholinergic. Post-ganglionic neurons join peripheral nerves and supply the end organs with noradrenergic nerve endings.

The preganglionic neurons receive excitatory and inhibitory synaptic inputs from the spinal cord, brain stem and other higher centres. There is a constant background discharge in these neurons called sympathetic tone. This is responsible for maintenance of tone in the smooth muscle of blood vessels, thereby maintaining blood pressure.

The sympathetic system tends to respond to stimuli as a whole system, uniformly throughout

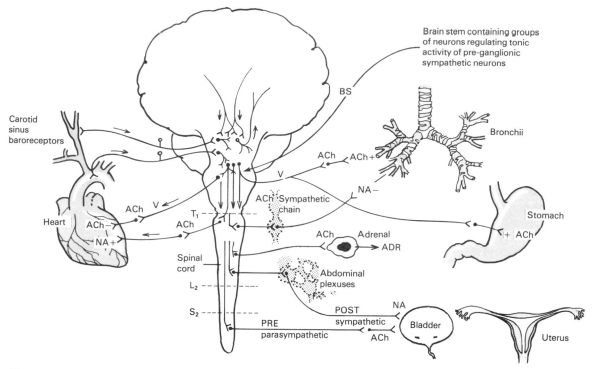

Fig. B.1 Schematic representation of the autonomic nervous system. ACh, Acetylcholine; NA, noradrenaline; ADR, adrenaline; V, vagus nerve; BS, brain stem; PRE, preganglionic neuron; POST, postganglionic neuron; + = stimulation; − = inhibition; Arrows indicate direction of traffic of nerve impulses

the body. All nerve endings discharge noradrenaline, with two known exceptions: sweat glands and blood vessels in voluntary muscle, which are cholinergic.

(b) Parasympathetic system

This has two main outflows from the central nervous system, one arising with cranial nerves and the other with sacral roots. Pre-ganglionic neurons are much longer than their equivalents in the sympathetic system but are also cholinergic. The ganglia are situated very close to or within the effector organs (e.g. Auerbach plexuses in the intestine). The post-ganglionic neurons are very short and release acetylcholine. The parasympathetic system tends to respond to stimuli in a more localised fashion. There is no evidence of parasympathetic tone regulating blood pressure.

(c) Innervation of effector organs

Most viscera are innervated by both sympathetic and parasympathetic systems; the effects of stimulation are usually antagonistic (e.g. sympathetic accelerates the heart, parasympathetic slows it; other examples are the pupil and bronchial smooth muscle). A few effectors receive innervation only from the sympathetic system, such as sweat glands and 'resistance' blood vessels in the skin and gut.

The description just given is an oversimplification of a very complex system both anatomically and functionally. Ganglia for example, far from being simple relay stations, are neuronal networks with more than one neurotransmitter involved. In addition to the neural pathways and neurotransmitters described above, there are other fibres innervating the same end organs which release other chemicals; some have a well-established role, but many of the newly described substances do not exhibit uniform effects in different species, and the relevance to human physiology is hypothetical. Examples are bradykinin, 5-hydroxytryptamine, enkephalin, substance P and vasoactive intestinal peptide (VIP).

Pharmacology

The natural transmitters adrenaline, dopamine and noradrenaline are often used therapeutically. A large number of synthetic drugs have been studied which mimic or block the effects of the natural transmitters at particular locations, depending upon the type of receptor present. Accordingly, they are designated agonists, partial agonists or competitive antagonists (Appendix A).

The neurotransmitters described in the autonomic nervous system are also present in the central nervous system. Consequently, drugs prescribed for peripheral effects should always be considered for their central effects as well, their state of ionisation in plasma dictating whether they cross the blood–brain barrier (Appendix A).

It makes sense to describe agonist and antagonist drugs in relation to the natural neurotransmitters.

(a) Cholinergic system

There are three types of peripheral cholinergic receptors, and there may be more within the central nervous system:

(1) Nicotinic cholinergic receptors occur at the neuromuscular synapse of voluntary muscle. Blocking drugs are discussed in Chapter 5. It is named 'nicotinic' after the first drug found to have agonist effects. Stimulation of this receptor produces depolarisation and contraction of voluntary muscle.

(2) Nicotinic receptors are also present at the synapses of both sympathetic and parasympathetic ganglia, and are also excitatory. The specific competitive antagonist drugs for this receptor are called ganglion-blockers and are used to lower blood pressure. Their effect is to reduce traffic of sympathetic

impulses which maintain tone in vascular smooth muscle. This class of drug is not used in ambulatory patients because of postural hypotension, but is used during anaesthesia to lower blood pressure (Chapter 8). The neuromuscular blocker tubocurarine has marked ganglion-blocking properties. Vecuronium and atracurium are much more specific for muscle receptors.

(3) Muscarinic receptors occur at parasympathetic nerve endings; muscarine mimics the action of acetylcholine at this receptor. Activation may be inhibitory (e.g. heart, arterioles, intestinal sphincters) or excitatory (salivary glands, bronchial and intestinal smooth muscle, bladder detrusor). Specific antagonists such as atropine are used in premedication and during surgery to suppress salivation and cardiac vagal reflexes (Chapter 2). Hyoscine crosses the blood–brain barrier easily, blocking central muscarinic receptors, causing amnesia and unconsciousness in high doses. Table B.1 lists examples of synthetic agonist and antagonist cholinergic drugs.

(b) Adrenergic system

There are two main types of adrenergic receptors, alpha and beta, which may co-exist in the same effector organ. Subtypes of these receptors, alpha-1 and 2 and beta-1 and 2, have been identified with the advent of specific blockers and agonists (Fig. B.2). They are distributed thoughout the body, including the central nervous system, and both types are activated by noradrenaline and adrenaline. Activation of alpha and beta receptors often has opposite physiological effects upon smooth muscle, such as in bronchi and in arterioles, a poorly understood phenomenon. Possibly regulation of synthesis of either type of receptor determines the relative effect of natural transmitters.

Classic examples of location of beta receptors are the heart (excitatory), uterus (inhibitory), bronchii (dilatation), arterioles supplying heart and muscle (dilatation), platelets (aggregation), and brown adipose tissue (heat production). Examples of alpha receptor location are the eye (mydriasis), skin and visceral arteries (con-

TABLE B.1. Synthetic drugs acting upon cholinergic receptors

Receptor type	Agonists	Antagonists
Nicotinic I (voluntary muscle)	nicotine, phenyl-trimethylammonium	tubocurarine, pancuronium alcuronium, gallamine, vecuronium, atracurium
Nicotinic II (autonomic ganglion)	nicotine, dimethyl-phenylpiperazinium	hexamethonium, pentolinium, trimetaphan
Muscarinic (heart, glands, smooth muscle)	muscarine, carbachol	atropine, hyoscine, glycopyrronium

striction), veins (constriction), and bladder sphincter (contraction). Alpha receptors have been identified in many structures without a complete understanding of their physiological role; such as the spinal cord, associated with pain pathways, in the brain stem associated with the control of blood pressure and temperature, and in human platelets.

Understanding of intracellular mechanisms mediating the step between activation of receptors and cellular response is still poor. Cyclic AMP is now well established as one intracellular mediator of excitatory phenomena triggered by beta agonists.

(1) *Alpha blockers* are no longer used as hypotensive agents in ambulatory patients because of postural effects and reflex tachycardia; phentolamine is used in cardiac surgery to lower blood pressure by a reduction in systemic vascular resistance (SVR).

Alpha agonists are more rarely used (e.g. phenylephrine to increase SVR in cardiopulmonary bypass).

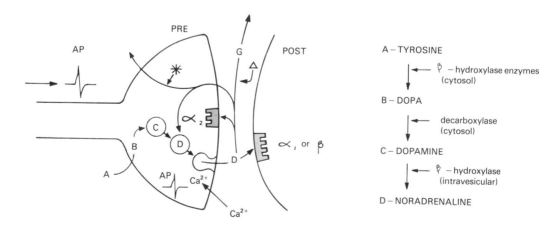

Fig. B.2 Noradrenergic synapse and steps in synthesis of noradrenaline. AP, Action potential; PRE, presynaptic terminal; POST, postsynaptic terminal; $\alpha_{1,2}$, alpha receptors; β, beta receptors; ◯, storage microvesicle containing noradrenaline; △, Catechol-O-methyltransferase (COMT); *, monoamine oxidase (MAO); G, normetadrenaline

(2) *Beta blocking* drugs have been extensively studied in recent years because of their application to long-term management of high blood pressure, dysrhythmias and anginal pain. The specificity of drugs for beta-1 and beta-2 receptors is far less marked than that seen between alpha and beta receptors. Asthmatic patients should never be given beta blockers; even drugs claimed as beta-1 specific may precipitate fatal bronchospasm.

Beta agonists are widely used as inotropic agents (e.g. isoprenaline), as bronchodilators in asthma (salbutamol) and to arrest labour in obstetrics (ritodrine). Salbutamol, claimed to be beta-2 specific, may cause severe tachycardia due to the presence of beta-2 receptors in the atria. There is evidence that beta receptors are also present in the central nervous system, such as medullary neurons regulating respiration and sympathetic tone.

(3) Some synthetic agonist drugs have both alpha and beta effects like the natural transmitters. They may act indirectly by promoting the release of noradrenaline (amphetamine) or by direct action on the receptor (metaraminol). Their state of ionisation in plasma determines how much crosses into the brain. Table B.2 gives examples of agonist and antagonist drugs.

(c) Dopaminergic system

Dopamine is the immediate precursor of noradrenaline, the step being catalysed by dopamine-beta-hydroxylase (present within the microvesicles of noradrenergic nerve terminals, Fig. B.2). Groups of central neurons lacking the enzyme secrete dopamine, such as found in pathways controlling voluntary movement (depletion causes Parkinson's disease), and vomiting reflexes (Chapter 5). Peripherally, dopamine receptors have been identified in the kidney (vasodilatation) and in the carotid body chemoreceptor (inhibition).

Dopamine infused at rates lower than 5 µg $kg^{-1} min^{-1}$ ('renal dose') specifically increases renal blood flow; at higher dosage it also has beta, and subsequently alpha effects. Examples of synthetic dopamine agonists are apomorphine (used rarely to induce vomiting) and bromocriptine. Dopamine blockers are used in psychiatric disorders (haloperidol), in neuroleptic anaesthesia (droperidol), and as antiemetics (metoclopramide).

(d) Other systems

There are other transmitter systems in the autonomic system, as stated earlier. A number of

TABLE B.2. Synthetic drugs acting upon adrenergic receptors

Receptor type	Agonists	Antagonists
alpha	phenylephrine methoxamine	phenoxybenzamine phentolamine tolazoline
beta 1 and 2	isoprenaline (1 and 2) salbutamol (2) ritodrine (2)	propranolol (1 and 2) practolol (1≫2) atenolol (1≫2) metoprolol (1≫2) butoxamine (2)
alpha and beta	ephedrine metaraminol amphetamine dobutamine	labetalol

drugs related to these systems are finding a place in clinical practice, such as ketanserin (5-hydroxytryptamine blocker), in the management of certain types of chronic limb pain.

Pharmacological Effects Unrelated to Receptors

Many other drugs act upon autonomic functions without directly interfering with receptors. They are mostly hypotensive agents.

(a) The action may be predominantly central, such as reserpine, which drops blood pressure by reducing sympathetic 'tone' centrally.

(b) Another group of drugs act at the pre-synaptic end of adrenergic terminals, by interfering with catecholamine synthesis (methyl-dopa), storage (reserpine), release (guanethidine) or re-uptake (desipramine), as outlined in Fig. B.2.

(c) The enzymatic breakdown of neurotransmitter may be inhibited, enhancing the local concentration of transmitter. Monoamine oxidase inhibitors slow down the breakdown of catecholamines, both peripherally and centrally; the latter effect may be beneficial in depression. Neostigmine acts by a similar mechanism on cholinergic terminals by inhibiting cholinesterase; it does not cross the blood–brain barrier (Appendix A). Another cholinesterase inhibitor, physostigmine, crosses easily into the brain; this is a useful feature to reverse central depressant effects of overdosage with hyoscine or tricyclic antidepressants.

(d) Finally, there is a group of drugs which act directly upon the smooth muscle cell. Examples are sodium nitroprusside and nitroglycerine whose hypotensive effects are initially mediated by relaxation of venous smooth muscle and at higher dosage by arteriolar dilatation as well. Hydrallazine also acts directly upon smooth muscle, with preference for the arteriolar side. Papaverine and theophylline are other examples of smooth muscle relaxants. The latter acts upon intracellular cyclic-AMP mediation of beta effects.

Tables of useful values and formulae

1 Biochemistry

(a) Blood

Adrenaline	0.54	nmol l^{-1}
Amylase	30–70	i.u. l^{-1}
Bicarbonate	20–32	mmol l^{-1}
Bilirubin (total)	3–20	μmol l^{-1}
Calcium total	2.1–2.7	mmol l^{-1}
ionised	1–1.2	mmol l^{-1}
Chloride	95–105	mmol l^{-1}
Cholesterol	9–25	mmol l^{-1}
Copper	13–24	nmol l^{-1}
Cortisol	170–700	nmol l^{-1}
Creatinine	45–120	μmol l^{-1}
Fibrinogen	1.5–4	g l^{-1}
Glucose (fasting)	3–6	mmol l^{-1}
Iodine	270–620	nmol l^{-1}
Iron	10–36	μmol l^{-1}
Ketones	40–80	μmol l^{-1}
Lactic acid	0.4–1.6	mmol l^{-1}
Lactic dehydrogenase	200–500	i.u. l^{-1}
Magnesium	0.7–1	mmol l^{-1}
Noradrenaline	2–3	nmol l^{-1}
Osmolality	280–295	mosmol kg^{-1}
Phosphatase acid	1–7	i.u. l^{-1}
alkaline	25–100	i.u. l^{-1}
Phosphate	0.8–1.4	mmol l^{-1}
Potassium	3.6–5.2	mmol l^{-1}
Protein total	60–80	g l^{-1}
albumin	35–55	g l^{-1}
globulin	25–35	g l^{-1}
Sodium	135–146	mmol l^{-1}
Thyroxine (T4)	60–150	nmol l^{-1}
Transaminase SGOT	0–30	i.u. l^{-1}
SGPT	0–24	i.u. l^{-1}
Urea	3.3–6.7	nmol l^{-1}
Zinc	0.5–1	mmol l^{-1}

(b) Urine

Adrenaline	0.05–085	μmol l^{-1}
Ammonium	18–60	mmol l^{-1}
Chloride	100–300	mmol l^{-1}
Glucose	0–11	mmol l^{-1}
Creatinine clearance	120	ml min^{-1}
Noradrenaline	30–600	nmol l^{-1}
Osmolality	200–1000	mosmol kg^{-1}
pH	4–8	
Phosphate	15–30	mmol l^{-1}
Potassium	30–100	mmol l^{-1}
Sodium	20–300	mmol l^{-1}
Specific gravity	1003–1030	

(c) Cerebrospinal fluid

Chloride	120–130	mmol l^{-1}
Glucose	2.2–5.5	mmol l^{-1}
Potassium	3–4	mmol l^{-1}
Protein	150–400	mg l^{-1}
Sodium	140	mmol l^{-1}
Lymphocytes	0–5 × 10^{-6}	
Osmolality	306	mosmol kg^{-1}
pH	7.3–7.35	
Pressure	7–15	cmH$_2$O
Protein	150–400	mg l^{-1}
Specific gravity	1007	
Volume	120–140	ml

(d) Electrolyte content of some body fluids

Fluid	Na$^+$	K$^+$	HCO$_3^-$ (mmol 1^{-1})	Cl$^-$	H$^+$
Bile	130	6	30–50	80	0.001–0.1
Diarrhoea	70	30	20–80	70	
Gastric	60	80	0	90	1–100
Small intestine	110	5	20–40	100	0.1–1
Sweat	50	10		45	

2 Haematology

Haemoglobin (Hb) male	14–16	$g\,dl^{-1}$
female	12–14	
Red blood cells male	5.4×10^{12}	l^{-1}
female........	4.8×10^{12}	l^{-1}
White blood cells	$4–11 \times 10^{+9}$	l^{-1}
Neutrophils	2.5–7	
Lymphocytes	1.5–7	
Monocytes	0.2–0.8	
Eosinophils	0–0.4	
Basophils	0–0.2	
Platelets	$150–400 \times 10^9$	l^{-1}
Packed cell volume (PCV) ...	0.40–0.47	

3 Respiratory Data

(a) Values at rest in normal adults, useful
for calculating ventilator settings

Alveolar ventilation (VA)	4–5	$l\,min^{-1}$
Minute volume (VE)	$100\,ml\,kg^{-1}\,min^{-1}$	$l\,min^{-1}$
Tidal volume (VT) ...	$8–10\,ml\,kg^{-1}\,min^{-1}$	$l\,min^{-1}$
Respiratory rate...........................	12–14	min^{-1}
Dead space (VD)		$2.2\,ml\,kg^{-1}$
Work of quiet breathing .... approx. 5		$J\,min^{-1}$
Airways resistance	1.6	$cmH_2O\,l^{-1}\,s^{-1}$
Total compliance	0.1	$1\,cmH_2O^{-1}$
Oxygen consumption (VO$_2$)	200–250	$ml\,min^{-1}$
Carbon dioxide production (VCO$_2$)		
....	150–200	$ml\,min^{-1}$
Respiratory quotient (VCO$_2$/VO$_2$) ...	0.8	

(b) Pulmonary function tests

Vital capacity (VC)	70	$ml\,kg^{-1}$
Forced expiratory volume in 1 s (FEV$_1$)	75% of VC	
Functional residual capacity (FRC)...	2.3–2.8	
Peak expiratory flow rate	400	$l\,min^{-1}$
Peak inspiratory flow rate	300	$l\,min^{-1}$
Total lung capacity (TLC)	5–6.5	
CO (DCO) diffusing capacity	2.3–2.7	$ml\,min^{-1}\,kP^{-1}$

(c) Alveolar gas equation

$$P_AO_{2'} = P_IO_2 - P_ACO_2/RQ$$
e.g. $13.3 = 20.0 - 5.3/0.8$ (kPa)

(d) Dead space equation

$$V_D/V_T = (P_ACO_2 - P_ECO_2)/P_ACO_2$$
$P_eCO_2 = PCO_2$ of mixed expired gas

4 Circulatory Values

(a) Regional blood flows in $ml\,min^{-1}$
and % of cardiac output (approximate values
for 65 kg adult)

Brain	700	14
Heart	200	4
Liver	1400	28
Kidneys	1200	24
Rest of the body	1500	30
Cardiac output	5000	100

(b) Cardiovascular pressures in mmHg

	Mean	Systolic	Diastolic
Right atrium (CVP)	0–8		
Left atrium (wedge)	6–12		
Right ventricle...........	12–16	14–33	0–7
Pulmonary artery	8–20	14–33	2–13
Left ventricle	40–60	100–150	2–12
Arterial	80–100	100–150	60–90

5 SI Units Conversion Factors

Pressure

1 mmHg	= 0.133 kPa	= 1.36 cmH$_2$O		
1 kPa	= 7.5 mmHg	= 10.2 cmH$_2$O	= 0.146 psi	
1 cmH$_2$O	= 0.098 kPa	= 0.735 mmHg		
1 psi	= 6.895 kPa	= 0.07 kg cm^{-2}		
1 Atm	= 101.3 kPa	= 760 mmHg	= 14.7 psi	= 1.03 kg cm^{-2}

Energy

1 J	= 0.239 cal
1 cal	= 4.187 J

6 Coagulation

Factors		Synthetised in liver	Vit K dependent	Consumed in clotting
I	Fibrinogen	+		+
II	Prothrombin	+	+	+
III	Thromboplastin	+		
IV	Calcium			
V	Accelerator globulin	+		+
VII	Pro-convertin	+	+	
VIII	Anti-haemophilic globulin			+
IX	Christmas factor (PTC)	+	+	
X	Stuart Power factor	+	+	
XI	Plasma thromboplastin antecedent (PTA)	+		
XII	Hageman factor	+		
XIII	Fibrin stabilising factor			

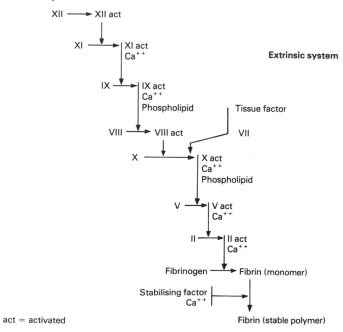

Intrinsic system

Extrinsic system

act = activated

7 Pharmacokinetic Data

Drug	Elimination half-life	Volume of distrib. ml kg^{-1}	Clearance ml min^{-1} kg^{-1}	pKa	% plasma protein binding
Alcuronium	3.3 h	360	1.34		
Alfentanyl	1.6 h	400	3.5		
Aminophylline	4 h	600	50		
Atenolol	6.3 h	70	1.3		
Aspirin	3 h	140	0.2	3.5	70–80
Atracurium	20 min	160	5.5		
Atropine	25 min	—	—	9.7	30–50
Bupivacaine	2.7 h	1000	0.58	8.1	95–98
Buprenorphine	5 h	2100	15		
Codeine	2 h			8.2	
Digoxin	40 h	3000	0.88		25
Droperidol	2 h			7.6	90
D-tubocurarine	3.8 h	600	2.25		67
Etomidate	3.5 h	3700		4.3	70
Fentanyl	3 h	4500	20	8.4	95
Frusemide	60 min	105	2.2	3.9	96
Gentamycin	3 h	250	GFR	2.8	10
Heparin	90 min	60	0.73		95
Hydrallazine	2.2 h	1600	10		87
Hydrocortisone	90 min		2.5		95
Insulin	2 h	48			
Isosorbide	30 min	1800	25		
Ketamine	2.2 h			7.5	
Lignocaine	100 min	1100	0.95	7.9	51
Lorazepam	15 h	1300	1.1	93	
Methohexitone	5 h	700		8	70–85
Metoclopramide	3 h	10			
Morphine	3 h	3200	15	7.9	35
Neostigmine	80 min	700	8.4		
Nitrazepam	29 h	2400	1		87
Nitroglycerine	1.8 h	340	2.2		
Pancuronium	2 h	300	1.8		88
Paracetamol	2 h	1000			
Pentazocine	2 h	3000	28	9.7	65
Perphenazine	20 h			7.8	
Pethidine	3.2 h	4500		8.7	50–70
Phenobarbitone	80 h	800	0.1	7.4	50–70
Phenytoin	20 h	600	8.4	8.3	89
Practolol	10 h	1500			<10
Prednisolone	3 h	480	3.6		90
Prilocaine			2.4		
Prochlorperazine	25 h			8.1	
Propranolol	4 h	3900	12	9.4	93
Salbutamol	3 h				
Suxamethonium	2 min				
Thiopentone	11 h	1400		7.6	60–97
Thyroxine	160 h		0.01		
Vecuronium	80 min	194	3		91
Verapamil	5 h		15		90
Warfarin	36 h	100	0.05	5.0	95–98

GLOSSARY

Alpha-adrenergic receptors Found in the radial muscle of the iris of the eye, in the blood vessels of skin and mucosae, blood vessels of cerebral, pulmonary and abdominal viscera circulations, platelets, hepatocytes, salivary glands, trigone and sphincter of the bladder, etc. Responses are usually excitatory but include inhibitory actions on intestinal musculature.

Amnesia Loss of memory following an injury or a drug. Can be retrograde (loss of memory of events occurring before injury/drug) or anterograde (loss of memory of events occurring after injury/drug).

Anaesthesia Absence of sensation. General anaesthesia means loss of all senses plus unconsciousness.

Analgesia Absence of pain sensation.

Analgesic Drug which reduces the perception of pain. There are central or narcotic analgesics such as morphine, and non-steroidal anti-inflammatory agents such as aspirin.

Antidepressants Drugs given to psychiatric patients to treat depression; mostly dibenzazepines of tricyclic structure (e.g. amitriptyline), rarely monoamine oxidase inhibitors (e.g. pargyline).

Antihypertensive Drug causing a fall of abnormally high arterial blood pressure (e.g. propranolol).

Antisialogogue Drugs which reduce secretion of saliva, such as atropine, hyoscine and glycopyrronium.

Beta-adrenergic receptors Found in the ciliary muscle of the eye, the heart, skeletal muscle, blood vessels, bronchial muscle, detrusor muscle of the bladder, uterus, etc. Responses are either inhibitory (blood vessels) or excitatory (heart, inotropic and chronotropic).

Bioavailability Fraction of oral dose of a drug reaching the systemic circulation after absorption and biotransformation in the liver. Bioavailability of 0.05 means that 5% of administered drug reaches the system circulation.

Biotransformation This refers to the chemical alteration of drugs by the body, mostly carried out in the liver; it may inactivate or activate the pharmacological properties of the drug.

Caudal Epidural anaesthesia administered through the sacro-coccygeal hiatus.

Cholinesterase Enzyme present in neuromuscular junction and other cholinergic synapses which breaks down acetylcholine.

Chronic pain Abnormal state in which pain has lost its protective value and has become the disease.

Chronotropic Drug affecting the rate of the heart beat.

Clearance of a drug Volume of blood cleared of drug per unit of time.

Compliance Volume change per unit of pressure exerted. When applied to the lung, the normal is $2 \, l \, kP^{-1}$ (200 ml cmH$_2$O^{-1}).

Core temperature Temperature of the hypothalamus; almost identical to the oesophagus or the heart.

CPAP Continous postive airways pressure. Applies to the spontaneously breathing subject; a constant pressure (up to 2 kPa) is applied during inspiration and expiration.

Cumulative effect Occurs with drugs often described as short acting because of fast redistribution to peripheral compartments but slow elimination; subsequent doses have a more prolonged effect.

Dissociative anaesthesia Anaesthesia produced by ketamine. In subanaesthetic doses there is loss of body image, hallucinations and intense analgesia.

Dysrhythmia (arrhythmia) Disorder of heart rhythm, e.g. tachycardia, atrial fibrillation.

131

Ectopic beats Heart beats produced by an action potential originating outside the sinus.

Elimination phase Refers to the fall in plasma concentration of a drug, after single injection, not due to distribution to peripheral compartments but due to biotransformation and excretion.

Enzyme induction Enhancing of mitochondrial metabolism of drugs (e.g. by chronic intake of alcohol).

Epidural or extradural space Space between dura mater and bone of the spinal canal, occupied by veins and fatty tissue.

Epidural anaesthesia/analgesia Local anaesthetic solution introduced into epidural space producing complete loss of sensation in affected dermatomes (anaesthesia) or only loss of pain (analgesia).

FIO$_2$ Fraction of inspired gas as oxygen. FIO$_2$ of 0.35 means 35% inspired oxygen.

Fresh gas flow Gas mixture moving from the anaesthetic machine into a gas delivery system.

Half-life (plasma) Time for the plasma concentration of a drug to fall by half.

IMV Intermittent mandatory ventilation; mechanical ventilation (IPPV) applied only to supplement the patient's natural breathing, usually during weaning off IPPV. It can vary from 10 to 90% of the total minute volume.

Induction of anaesthesia Administration of a drug causing loss of consciousness (e.g. thiopentone).

Inhalational anaesthesia Anaesthesia administered via the lung epithelium by means of gases or vapours.

Inotropic Drug causing a change in myocardial contractility. Positive inotropes stimulate and negative inotropes depress.

IPPV Intermittent positive pressure ventilation.

Maintenance of anaesthesia Administration of drug or combination of drugs which maintain a state of surgical anaesthesia for an indeterminate period of time.

MMV Mandatory minute volume; mechanical ventilation (IPPV) applied only if the patient fails to achieve a pre-set minute volume. Used in weaning of IPPV.

Monoamine oxidase inhibitors Antidepressant agents acting by inhibiting monoamine oxidase in central pathways, but also inhibiting the enzyme peripherally.

Nerve block Application of local anaesthetic around a peripheral nerve causing temporary interruption of conduction of nerve impulses.

Neuroleptanaesthesia Combination of narcotic analgesic (usually fentanyl) with droperidol, suitable to supplement N$_2$O/NMB anaesthetic technique.

Neuromuscular blockers Drugs which specifically block the neuromuscular synapse (e.g. tubocurarine).

Opiate/opioid Drug derived from opium. Opioid is a term often used for a drug with powerful analgesic and hypnotic action.

PEEP Positive end expiratory pressure, applied during IPPV.

Recovery of anaesthesia Recuperation of consciousness and protective physiological reflexes following the discontinuation of an anaesthetic.

Reducing valve A device to reduce a high pressure from a gas cylinder (e.g. 10,000 kPa) to a lower pressure of e.g. 400 kPa.

Respiration The process of gaseous exchange of oxygen and carbon dioxide which occurs between the tissues, blood and the external environment and includes the process of ventilation (q.v.)

Rotameter Flowmeter of the variable orifice type, designed for the continuous monitoring of gas or liquid flows. The position of a bobbin 'floating' inside a vertical tube of increasing internal cross-section area is proportional to flow.

Shock State of circulatory failure causing diminished oxygen delivery to tissues.

SI Unit Systeme internationale d'unités.

Spinal (subarachnoid) anaesthesia Local anaesthetic solution injected directly into the CSF.

Topical anaesthesia Anaesthesia obtained by direct application of drugs to mucosal, serosal or skin surfaces, e.g. eye, trachea.

T-piece Piece of tubing with a side port to deliver the fresh gas flow to a gas delivery system.

Ventilation (human) Movement of gas in and out of the lung.

Volatile agent Anaesthetic agent in liquid form at room temperature, and administered as a vapour to the lung.

Volume of distribution Volume calculated by dividing the (i.v.) dose of drug given by the initial plasma concentration.

Multiple choice questionnaire

Answers will be found at the end of the questionnaire. Each question relates to a chapter in the book (e.g. question 1 is based on topics covered in Chapter 1) and each branch should be answered as 'true' or 'false'.

1 The following are true or false:

(a) nitrous oxide was the first anaesthetic to receive wide acceptance
(b) spinal anaesthesia was first demonstrated at the turn of the century
(c) poliomyelitis epidemic triggered major developments in breathing apparatus
(d) halothane superseded ether just before the Second World War
(e) thiopentone was introduced to clinical use by Bier in 1900

2A A 71-year-old emphysematous patient is admitted for prostatectomy under GA. The following are important predictive factors (in history/examination), regarding his recovery after surgery:

(a) FEV_1 <50% of predicted
(b) inability to walk 50 metres on the flat
(c) $PaCO_2$ > 8 kPa (60 mmHg) and PaO_2 < 8 kPa
(d) presence of peripheral cyanosis
(e) presence of clubbing

2B Acceptable premedication for a 20 kg 5-year-old child admitted for tonsillectomy includes:

(a) papaveretum 12.5 mg and hyoscine 0.8 mg
(b) promethazine 75 mg orally
(c) trimeprazine 80 mg orally

(d) pethidine 20 mg promethazine 12.5 mg i.m.
(e) diazepam 10 mg orally

3. Advantages of the 'circle' over a non-rebreathing anaesthetic circuit include:

(a) reduction of theatre pollution due to reduced fresh gas flow
(b) increased humidification of inspired gas
(c) economy due to reduced fresh gas flow
(d) reduced apparatus resistance due to the presence of 1-way valves
(e) reduction of contamination due to bactericidal effect of soda lime

4A When performing endotracheal intubation:

(a) a tube of size 9 is suitable for the average adult male
(b) a tube of size 8, means that its external diameter is 8 mm
(c) the neck should be extended to optimally align the larynx
(d) the blade of the laryngoscope should be initially directed towards the right tonsil
(e) the cuffed portion of the tube should lie at the level of the cords to prevent aspiration of gastric contents

4B Important aspects of preventing accidental removal of an i.v. cannula include:

(a) shaving the skin to allow greater tape adhesion
(b) the diameter of the cannula
(c) shielding the giving set from potential sources of pulling
(d) tensile strength of the tape
(e) use of luer locking devices between cannula and giving set

133

4C When measuring blood pressure, the following statements are true or false:

(a) direct measurement is usually performed through a cannula in the radial artery
(b) palpated systolic pressure is usually 5–10 mmHg above that found by auscultation
(c) automated machines are usually based on the principles of oscillometry
(d) when using an oscillotonometer diastolic pressure is obtained by noting a sudden increase in oscillations
(e) in the operating theatre an oscillotonometer is preferred because it is more accurate than sphygmomanometry

5A The following factors increase the rate of rise of alveolar anaesthetic partial pressure (gases and volatile agents):

(a) increased minute volume of ventilation
(b) increased concentration of gas or vapour
(c) increased cardiac output
(d) increased blood solubility of the anaesthetic
(e) increased venous partial pressure of anaesthetic

5B Intravenous induction of anaesthesia is preferred to inhalational because:

(a) causes less side effects
(b) there is no hangover effect
(c) blood pressure and cardiac output are better maintained
(d) there is less danger of respiratory obstruction
(e) it is quicker

5C The following statements are true or false:

(a) acetylcholine is destroyed at the neuromuscular junction by pseudocholinesterase
(b) suxamethonium is a non-depolarising neuromuscular blocker
(c) tubocurarine may cause hypotension due to alpha blockade
(d) atracurium and vecuronium are the shortest-acting competitive blockers

(e) suxamethonium is the agent of choice in burn patients

5D When using lignocaine as a local analgesic:

(a) the maximum dose is 600 mg of the plain solution in a 60 kg patient
(b) 10 ml of 4% solution contains 40 mg
(c) adrenaline is added to increase the duration of action
(d) it should be used as a 2% solution for Bier's block (i.v. regional analgesia)
(e) in overdose CNS toxicity is common

5E The following statements are true or false:

(a) pentazocine is the analgesic of choice for myocardial infarction pain
(b) pethidine should be administered at greater than 4 hourly intervals for postoperative pain
(c) domperidone may be preferred to metoclopramide as it has less tendency to cross the blood–brain barrier
(d) the transmitter involved at the chemoreceptor trigger zone is noradrenaline
(e) the partial agonist analgesics are less likely to cause addiction than agonists such as morphine

6A The normal daily water and electrolyte requirements of a 60 kg adult are:

(a) 30–40 ml kg^{-1} of fluid
(b) 3 mmol kg^{-1} of potassium
(c) 1–2 mmol kg^{-1} of sodium
(d) calculated as 1500 ml + 20 ml for every kg above 20 kg
(e) 2300 ml of dextrose saline with a K$^+$ content of approximately 20 mmol 1^{-1}

6B The following statements are true or false:

(a) the blood volume of a 5 kg baby is 800 ml
(b) when estimating blood loss by weighing swabs, 1 g of excess weight is roughly equal to 1.25 ml of blood
(c) 85% of the population are Rhesus positive because they contain the Rhesus antigen
(d) rapid infusions of blood should be warmed, primarily to avoid excessive cooling of the liver

(e) a very low platelet count is one of the indicators of disseminated intravascular coagulation

7 The following are common complications during anaesthesia:

(a) hypotension following induction in the volume-depleted patient
(b) dysrhythmias during maintenance with volatile agents and spontaneous respiration
(c) headaches following a balanced anaesthetic technique
(d) headaches following spinal analgesia
(e) sore throat following mask anaesthesia

8 In assessing a patient for day case surgery, it is essential that:

(a) the patient is accompanied home after the procedure
(b) short-acting anaesthetic agents are used if possible
(c) a heavy premedication is administered if the patient is nervous
(d) a blood sample for Hb is always taken
(e) the patient is starved for at least 2 hours prior to the procedure

9 When assessing an arterial blood gas result:

(a) a raised $PaCO_2$ always indicates that the patient has abnormal lung function
(b) an acute increase in $PaCO_2$ of 1.3 kPa (10 mmHg) results in a fall in pH of 0.1 unit
(c) a negative base excess suggests that the patient is alkalotic
(d) bicarbonate should not be given if the $PaCO_2$ is raised
(e) a PO_2 of less than 4 kPa (30 mmHg) usually confirms that the sample was venous and not arterial

10 The pathophysiological effects of IPPV include:

(a) decreased cardiac output
(b) pneumothorax
(c) hepatic failure
(d) hypotension, especially in the volume-depleted patient
(e) poor intestinal function

11 The following statements are true or false:

(a) supraglottic infection causing airway obstruction is usually due to laryngotracheobronchitis
(b) an extrathoracic obstruction results in an inspiratory stridor
(c) during therapy, an adequate PaO_2 to aim for is 8 kPa (60 mmHg) in a patient with chronic respiratory failure
(d) previous history regarding exercise tolerance is essential in determining the place of IPPV in the treatment of respiratory failure in a chronic bronchitic
(e) a paediatric patient with airway obstruction should always have a lateral neck X-ray to exclude epiglottitis as the cause

12 During oxygen therapy:

(a) a low flow oxygen mask (e.g. MC) is suitable for the bronchitic patient without CO_2 retention
(b) an air entrainment device (e.g. Vickers) giving a fixed concentration of oxygen is essential in the treatment of patients with hypoxic ventilatory drive
(c) an FIO_2 of 0.4 should not be exceeded for long periods (days) due to the possibility of oxygen toxicity
(d) an FIO_2 of 0.3 should result in a PaO_2 of at least 20 kPa (150 mmHg) in the normal subject
(e) with a low flow mask (e.g. MC) a fall in ventilation results in an increase of FIO_2

13 In the patient suffering from septic shock:

(a) tissue perfusion may be decreased despite a high cardiac output due to shunting of blood through capillary beds
(b) oxygen therapy (FIO_2 0.4) is indicated
(c) endothelial damage results primarily from severe hypotension
(d) lung damage is always secondary to oxygen toxicity
(e) a satisfactory mean arterial blood pressure is 60 mmHg

14A The following statements are true or false:

(a) cardiac output is always low in cardiac failure
(b) preload is a minor determinant of cardiac output
(c) basal crepitations suggest that there is an element of right heart failure
(d) cardiac oxygen demand is increased by an elevated heart rate
(e) inotropes are the treatment of choice for a patient with a high PCWP and LVSWI.

14B When measuring CVP

(a) there should be no respiratory fluctuation of the column of fluid
(b) zero is taken as the level of the manubriosternal joint
(c) the catheter should be inserted as far as the superior vena cava or right atrium
(d) a low value suggests volume depletion
(e) left heart failure may give misleading results

15 A suitable 24 hour parenteral feeding regime for a post-operative patient (weight 60 kg) includes:

(a) 10,000 kJ (2400 kCal)
(b) 60 g of nitrogen as amino acids
(c) 240 g of lipid
(d) 150 mmol of magnesium
(e) 60 mmol of potassium

16 The following statements are true or false:

(a) burn injury has very serious metabolic implications because the skin is the largest organ in the body
(b) a convenient way of estimating the size of a burn area is the 'rule of nines'
(c) there is no point in applying gastric lavage for atropine poisoning as it increases gastric emptying
(d) there is no specific antidote for paracetamol poisoning
(e) apomorphine is a suitable emetic for children

17 The sensation of pain:

(a) travels in the B and C fibres
(b) is modified in some patients by antidepressants
(c) can be inhibited by naturally occurring opioid peptides
(d) can be inhibited by a central inhibitory pathway
(e) in malignancy is often best treated initially by a combination of opiates and NSAIDS

18 The following statements are true or false:

(a) adrenaline may be used to prolong the duration of a ring block
(b) pneumothorax is a complication of intercostal nerve block
(c) during Bier's block, the cannula must be inserted as close as possible to the antecubital fossa
(d) comprehensive resuscitation facilities should always be available where Bier's blocks are performed
(e) headache occurs in at least 10% of patients following a spinal anaesthetic

APP A. The following statements are true or false:

(a) pharmacokinetics is what the body does to the drug
(b) pharmacodynamics is what the drug does to the body
(c) clearance is the amount of drug excreted in unit time
(d) zero order kinetics states that a constant amount of the drug is metabolised in unit time, regardless of its plasma concentration
(e) in the presence of a high concentration of pure agonist, a partial agonist behaves as if it were an antagonist

APP B. The following result specifically from beta receptor stimulation:

(a) bronchodilatation
(b) bradycardia
(c) arteriolar constriction
(d) sweating
(e) increased cardiac contractility

Answers

A maximum score of 145 (29 × 5) is possible. The average student should be able to score approximately 70 after the first reading of the text.
Complete explanation for each question is to be found in the text.

Explanation of abbreviations and terms used in the test:

e.g. – for example; i.v. – intravenous; i.m. – intramuscular; CNS – central nervous system; GA – general anaesthetic; PCWP – pulmonary capillary wedge pressure; CVP – central venous pressure; LVSWI – left ventricular stroke work index; NSAIDs – non-steroidal anti-inflammatory drugs; IPPV – intermittent positive pressure ventilation; MC – Mary Caterall; fresh gas flow – refers to gas mixture delivered by the anaesthetic machine.

Answers:

1 F,T,T,F,F	2A T,T,T,F,F	2B F,F,T,T,F
3 T,T,T,F,F	4A T,F,F,T,F	4B T,F,T,T,F
4C T,F,T,F,F	5A T,T,F,F,T	5B F,F,F,F,T
5C F,F,F,T,F	5D F,F,T,F,T	5E F,F,T,F,T
6A T,F,T,T,T	6B F,T,T,F,T	7 T,T,F,T,F
8 T,T,F,F,F	9 F,T,F,T,T	10 T,T,F,T,T
11 F,T,T,T,F	12 T,T,T,T,T	13 T,T,F,F,T
14A F,F,F,T,F	14B T,T,T,T,F	15 T,F,F,F,T
16 T,T,F,F,F	17 F,T,T,T,T,	18 F,T,F,T,F

APPA T,T,F,T,T APP B T,F,F,F,T

Suggested further reading

Chapters 1 and 2
Churchill-Davidson, H. C. (1984). *A Practice of Anaesthesia*, 5th edn. Lloyd-Luke, London.

Chapter 3
Ward, C. S. (1985). *Anaesthetic Equipment, Physical Principles and Maintenance*. 2nd edn. Baillière Tindall, Eastbourne.

Chapter 5 and Appendix A
Calvey, T. N. and Williams, N. E. (1982). *Principles of Pharmacology for Anaesthetists*. Blackwell Scientific Publications, Oxford.
Vickers, M. D., Schneider, H. and Wood-Smith, F. G. (1984). *Drugs in Anaesthetic Practice*, 6th edn. Butterworths, London.

Chapters 6 and 9
Willatts, S. (1982). *Lecture Notes on Fluid and Electrolyte Balance*. Blackwell Scientific Publications, Oxford.

Marshall, M. and Bird, T. (1983). *Blood Loss and Replacement*. Edward Arnold, London.

Chapters 7 and 8
Atkinson, R. S., Rushman, G. B. and Lee, J. A. (1982). *A Synopsis of Anaesthesia*, 9th edn. Wright PSG, Bristol.

Chapters 9–16
Shoemaker, W. C. (1984). *Textbook on Critical Care Medicine*. W. B. Saunders, Philadelphia.

Chapter 17
Wall, P. and Melzack, R. (1982). *The Challenge of Pain*. Penguin Books, Harmondsworth.

Chapter 18
Eriksson, E. (1979). *Illustrated Handbook in Local Anaesthesia*, 2nd end. Lloyd-Luke, London.

Appendix B
Appenzeller, O. (1982). *The Autonomic Nervous System*, 2nd end. Elsevier, Amsterdam.

Index